CONGRUENT EXE

How To Make Weight Training
Easier on Your Joints

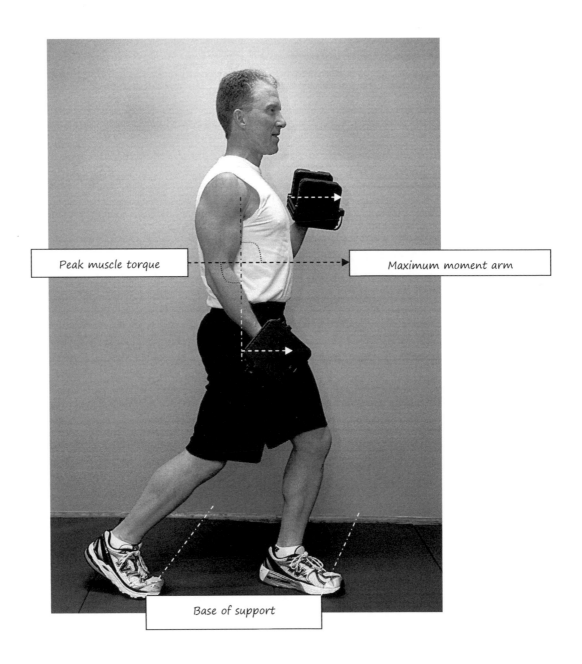

Peak muscle torque

Maximum moment arm

Base of support

Bill DeSimone

This book is intended as a reference volume only, not a medical manual. The information given here is designed to help you make informed decisions about your health. It is not intended as a substitute for any treatment that may have been prescribed by your doctor.

All forms of exercise pose some inherent risks. The reader is advised to take full responsibility for their safety and know their limits. Before practicing the exercises in this book, be sure the equipment is well maintained, and do not take risks beyond your level of experience, aptitude, training, and fitness. As with all fitness programs, you should get your doctor's approval before beginning. If you suspect that you have a medical problem, you are urged to seek competent medical help.

Mention of specific companies, organizations, or authorities in this book does not imply endorsement by the author or publisher, nor does mention of specific companies, organizations, or authorities imply that they endorse the book, the author, or the publisher.

Although all the following material is useful to beginners as well as more experienced trainees, **Congruent Exercise** is not intended to be an introduction to weight training. The author assumes the reader is familiar with the fundamentals of weight training: what reps, sets, barbells, dumbbells, etc. are, and common names for the various exercises.

User assumes all risk for performing the exercises described in this work. Use of the material constitutes an agreement not to bring any lawsuit or action for injury caused by performing the exercises illustrated in this material.

DeSimone, William S.

Congruent Exercise: how to make weight training easier on your joints/ William S. DeSimone

CONTENTS

ACKNOWLEDGMENTS

To Greg Anderson (Ideal Exercise, "Seattle's home for high intensity training", not the more notorious one), Fred Hahn(Serious Strength NYC, Slow Burn), and Doug McGuff(Body by Science, Ultimate Exercise), whose early support for Moment Arm Exercise gave me instant credibility.

To Bo Railey and Exercise Inc., Karen Heffernan and Strength Club, Anthony Johnson and the 21 Convention, Chris Highcock and Conditioning Research, Luke Carlson and Discover Strength, and Adam Zickerman and Inform Fitness, who provided additional audiences for the approach.

To all the forum posters, (especially on Dr. Darden's and John Little's boards), You Tube subscribers, emailers, video review clients, conference attendees, and "regular guys" and women, whose continuing interest confirms the need for this approach.

To Jeff Granit for the original photography. Thanks, Jeff!
To Laura Jackson for the digital magic. Thanks, Laura!

Dedicated to Linda, Matt, and Amanda

Preface

You would think that with all the exercise options available today, it should go without saying that what you do to get in shape actually had some relationship with proper muscle and joint function.

You would think that for all the avenues of exercise information—the websites, magazines, certifications, academic departments, etc.-- that someone would regularly compare a biomechanics textbook to what human joints and muscles are subject to in exercise, and identify any questionable practices.

You would think that for as many times as we see the words "functional" and "biomechanically-correct" and "safe and effective", that there would never be any injuries or problems resulting from exercise, and that everyone indulging in it would have a stronger, pain-free, injury-free body as a result.

You might think that, but it's not true. There have been several high-profile injuries to top athletes in the weight room, all of which were easily preventable, and worse, easily predictable, to anyone with even a passing familiarity with biomechanics. But it's not just catastrophic events happening to high level athletes, who might be willing to accept more risk in hope of a substantial reward. Much of what we find in commercial exercise subjects the joints and muscles to strains that simply cannot be met, over time, by human anatomy; and no, it's not a question "working through" or "getting used to it". Many of the joint movements and loading patterns found in classic, free-weight bodybuilding, so-called "functional training", and machine designs are guilty of this.

And while not as dramatic as the athletes' injuries, over time, this strain can contribute to a long list of chronic conditions, such as back and knee pain, impingements, tendinitis, bursitis, ruptures, tears. Yes, people who don't lift weights also get these conditions, but the wear and tear of a lifetime that leads to those conditions is already there. Why add to it with poorly designed exercises?

Of course, the long-term detriment will only be there if you stick with it. How many people drop out of exercise because their results don't measure up? How many people get frustrated, because they don't continue to improve as they've been led to believe? So they read another website and try another scheme, or they go the supplement and ergogenic aids route, which can lead to all sorts of confusion and frustration and all that entails.

Wow. Rereading the preceding paragraphs, it may be hard to believe that I'm actually a huge advocate of weight training and exercise. I've been using weights myself for almost 40 years (I should be HUGE). I started as a personal trainer in 1983, I've been certified by two of the major organizations, and I train clients in my own studio. I've competed …well, maybe "participated" is more accurate…I've participated in bodybuilding, triathlon, inline skating, martial arts, softball, and the usual sports.

And boy, have I inflicted some damage on myself. Nothing particularly life-threatening, a back ache here, a ruptured biceps there, a ruptured triceps also there, a chronic sore shoulder, but enough to get my attention. So a few years ago, I put aside my old muscle magazines and trade paperbacks and firmly held beliefs, and dove into texts on biomechanics and anatomy and kinesiology and simple machines. Most of those texts aren't written with working out in mind; they are more like reference texts.

I eventually settled on a pattern of starting with a basic conventional exercise, looking at the relevant anatomy and movements, and then modifying the exercise to match textbook muscle-and joint- function. I tried the exercises on myself, and where appropriate, on clients, until I arrived at the set of exercises illustrated here. I began to present the material, first in a manual called **Moment Arm Exercise**, then at in-services, conferences, and most recently on You Tube, hopefully refining the presentation so that the concepts to follow are clear and accurate enough for you to use in the gym tomorrow.

A few disclaimers. First, I'm a trainer. I'm not a physiologist, or a doctor, or a mechanical engineer, or a biomedical engineer, or a kinesiologist, or physical therapist...you get the drift. I'm trying to apply what appears to be proper muscle and joint function, as laid out in those texts, to getting another human being to lift a heavy thing for health purposes. So I may sacrifice the precision of a reference text in labeling or describing, in order to relate what to do in the gym now. Hopefully, we gain in clarity what I give up in precision. If you need the exact nomenclature, well, that's what bibliographies are for.

Second, I'm not the Reality-Show-Trainer-Star-type. I'm not afraid of, or opposed to, hard physical work as part of getting in shape, but I do prefer to avoid unintended consequences. I've heard people say that injuries are the price you pay to get in great shape. That's silly and self-defeating. The price you pay is the time you spend doing it, that you could be doing something else. Setting yourself up for a back or shoulder injury (or worse), now or in the future, is a heavy price to pay, especially when the information to avoid it is easily available now, and when the connection between the risk and reward is speculative at best.

Finally, to be clear on the context: Weight training has undeniable benefits. It can give shape and strength to our muscles, and make the physical parts of our day easier. It can help prevent injury, and keep us mobile and functional as we age. It can help our mood and self-esteem, and dozens of other measures.

It can also crush spines, throats, and jaws; tear rotator cuffs, rupture biceps, quadriceps, and other muscles; and combined with everything else in life, contribute to chronic joint problems. And it can be frustrating and lead to a number of dead ends.

Both the pros and cons are true; fortunately, it's not an either/or situation. You can get all the benefits of weight training, without the risk and frustration, by applying the appropriate joint movements, postures, moment arms, i.e. biomechanics , to your exercises. And you'll be able to apply this anywhere, whether you are surrounded by the most current, high tech, selectorized machines, or sewer plates on a rusty bar, or doing chin-ups on a tree, because the one constant is your body and biomechanics.

Here's how.

Bill DeSimone

Many months in 2010 and 11

Introduction

Congruent Exercise offers a unique, biomechanics-based approach to weight training. By putting safe muscle and joint function first, and then designing the exercises to fit that, the goal is to get all the benefits of weight training, without any injuries or chronic conditions, over years of training.

Much of today's exercise scene is based on performance: competing with others in a group workout, setting a personal record in a lift, finishing a machine circuit in a faster time. And you certainly can get in shape this way, but frequently at a physical cost. This might be a perfectly valid approach to a sports competition, for which you'll make some short-term sacrifice for the larger goal of winning the event. While there certainly is a value to peaking for a specific event, by definition, it's not training that can last.

I'm more interested in the long haul. You could use this material in a peaking strategy; although in all honestly, if you look at the training programs of champion athletes and fitness celebrities, they are far more extreme than what you'll find here. I'm looking at weight training as a regular activity, every week, for a lifetime, to get whatever benefits you can for as long as you can. Aching shoulders, backs, and knees, not to mention more serious injuries, tend to discourage that. And since many of those aches, pains, and injuries come from the disconnect between Biomechanics and Exercise, it's a pretty direct fix.

You may be surprised that many of the joint motions you're used to seeing in conventional exercise, contradict safe joint motions as described in biomechanics textbooks. Part of that comes from compromised sports, dance, and martial arts movements working their way into exercise. Part of it comes from the visceral appeal of exercise ("no pain, no gain") and associating "feel" with benefit, even if what you're feeling is strain. While popular exercise concerns itself with bigger biceps and ripped abdomens, academic biomechanics are working on joint replacements and prosthetics. (Where ARE their priorities?) This leaves a huge gap, where basic biomechanics could be applied to exercises, taking some of the material from academia and dropping it into the gym where people might be able to use it earlier in life. **Congruent Exercise** is intended to do just that.

I have presented much of the first 5 chapters previously in conferences, in Orlando for Anthony Johnson's 21 Convention in 2010, and in Minneapolis for Luke Carlson's HIT Resurgence in 2011. Video is available on You Tube and as part of larger packages through both Anthony and Luke. This manual elaborates on that material, and adds 20 exercises demonstrating the appropriate joint patterns, using both commercial equipment and dumbbells, bodyweight, and light gear.

1. Avoiding The Tragic "Accident": Biomechanics You Need To Know

The absolute first priority for anyone training with weights should be to avoid a catastrophic injury. That should be obvious, but consider the following:

- In 1972, Muscular Development magazine reported on a Pennsylvania man, found dead in his home, on his bench press, with the bar across his throat. He apparently missed his lift, the bar landed on his chest, and rolled to his throat, strangling him.
- In 2002, Flex magazine reported on a competitive bodybuilder, performing a barbell squat with 675 pounds for a photo shoot. As he bent his knees, he lost control of the descent, landing on his knees, then falling backwards with the weight. His quadriceps and patellar ligaments were torn, resulting in multiple surgeries, months of rehab, and putting his ability to walk at risk.
- In 2003, Club Industry magazine reported on a lawsuit brought by a man using a Smith machine for squats. He wasn't able to control the descent of the bar, the machine did not have bottom stops, and so his spine was crushed between the bar and the floor, leaving him quadriplegic.
- In 2007, a college football player, after performing the step-up exercise with 185 pounds on a bar across his shoulders, twisted an ankle returning the bar to the rack, and fell with the barbell. He suffered injuries to his spine and, again, his ability to walk was put at risk.
- In 2009, a college football player, bench pressing 275 pounds with a spotter, missed the lift, dropped the bar on his throat, and had to have 3 emergency surgeries on his vocal cords, adam's apple and neck.

These instances, which involved a range of trainees from guys working out at home and in commercial gyms to high level athletes, are always reported as tragic, freak accidents. And it is tragic that these people suffered life-altering injuries doing something that was supposed to be life-enhancing, and that clearly they weren't intending on getting injured, so in that sense, these are accidents.

But what is especially tragic is that even though these are standard exercises, the injuries they could cause are predictable and preventable. An analysis of even the most fundamental biomechanics suggests that the "freak" occurrence is when you push these exercises hard and *don't* get hurt. Squats and bench press are especially dangerous, because your spine, and your throat, face, and jaw are between the barbell and gravity. Here are the biomechanics you need to know to avoid a catastrophic injury:

- Free weights "get heavier" as you bend.
- You can lower more weight than you can lift.
- The bones and muscles of the spine aren't suited for top-heavy loads.
- Balancing on one leg or a split stance relies on small muscles of the hip and deep muscles of the spine.
- Putting the weight back relies on much smaller muscles than the ones that lifted it.

Free weights "get heavier" as you bend.

Anyone who has done a squat or bench press with a barbell knows this to be true. Put the bar on your shoulders to start the squat, and while you're standing with your knees and back straight, the weight is manageable. Same with the bench press, as you take the bar off the rack and your elbows are straight. As soon as you break the lock at the knees and elbows, the weight starts to get heavier, becoming heaviest the closer you get to the bottom.

But it's not "heavier"; it's the same barbell. Something changed from lockout to sticking point, but it isn't the weight. It's the moment arm, or the lever through which the weight acts.

The clearest way to demonstrate Moment Arm is with a Seesaw. Walk up one side of a seesaw (for demonstration purposes only, don't try this at home) and stand directly over the axle. No matter what

you weigh, conceivably, you could balance both sides of the plank off the ground, because your weight is directly over the axis. But if you take one step to either side, or even shift your weight, the plank tips. By moving your weight away from the axis, you introduce a moment arm, making your same weight "heavier".

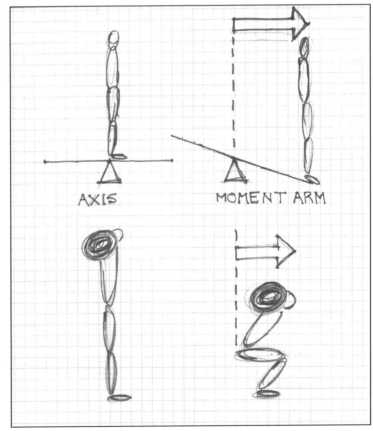

AXIS   MOMENT ARM

With the barbell squat and bench press, when the weight is directly over your joints, it's the same as standing over the axle. "Lockout" is the same as no moment arm: the axes are in line with the weight. As you break lockout in the squat, and your hips move back, it has the same effect as stepping to the side on the seesaw. Instead of the weight walking away from the axis (the seesaw), the axis is moving

2

away from the weight. Either way, a moment arm is created, and the weight gets "heavier".

The moment arms in the barbell bench press are less visual, but as you lower, the weight moves away from directly over the shoulders and elbows. It's easier to see with dumbbells. Since hand width is fixed on a barbell, as the elbows bend, they also move away, so you get moment arms created at both sets of joints. With barbells or dumbbells, the weights get harder to handle as they approach the bench presser.

This easy-to-hard pattern is in play at all weight levels, but is obviously more of a concern at maximum efforts. With a light enough weight, you could conceivably throw the weight off or push it to the side if you run into trouble. As you approach your maximum, this becomes less of an option, and if you're in a smith machine, it's not an option. Practically, this means you could guess wrong about your capability, put too much weight on the bar, start out ok, and then only realize, too late, that it's too heavy. So the conventional squat and bench press with a barbell moves from easy-to-hard, mechanically. There's also a muscular aspect.

You can lower more weight than you can lift.

Muscles are commonly described as having three levels of strength. Positive strength comes from the shortening of muscle (a "concentric contraction"); an example of which is lifting a weight. A higher level of strength is isometric ("static contraction"), where the muscle exerts effort to hold its' position. The highest level is "negative" strength ("eccentric contraction"), which comes from allowing the muscle to lengthen under control.

Practically, in the gym, this has several applications. Generally, if you've lifted a weight ten times, and can't complete number eleven, you could stop your set at ten. Or, you could begin rep 11, stall during the rep, and hold that position for as long as you can, extending your set. And if you have attentive training partners, they can then lift the weight for you, so you can lower it under control, extending the set even further.

It could also go the other way ("negative training"), where you deliberately pick a weight heavier than you could lift and just do the lowering portion of the set. If you can't do a chin up, for example, you could climb to the top, and only do the lowering portion of the rep; which obviously allows you to work those muscles better than not doing any chin ups.

The issue with the squat and bench press, however, is if you don't realize the weight is too heavy.

For exercises where you lift, first, if you pick too heavy a weight, you know right away that you can't do the rep. Put 500 pounds on a bar and try to deadlift it. Put 200 pounds on a bar and try to curl it. You'll know right away that the weight is too heavy, and generally stop before anything bad happens.

With the squat and the bench press, you start at lockout, the mechanically easiest part. You're also starting with the lowering phase, where you can handle more weight than you can lift or hold. You might actually be able to start the squat with the same 500 pounds you walked away from on the deadlift, and you might be able to lower it under control; but if you realize it's too heavy, you may not be able to lift it, and you may not be able to stop it. The same aspects of muscle strength that allow you to extend your set, and to practice chin-ups, even to walk down steps with little effort, can cause real problems on the squat and bench.

Starting at lockout and doing the negative first apply to both the squat and bench press. The squat has the added complication of involving the spine.

The bones and muscles of the spine aren't suited for top-heavy loads.

Take a look at the human skeleton, the spine in particular, preferably a rear or side view. Starting at the pelvis and looking towards the head, we see three sections of vertebrae: 5 lumbar, 12 thoracic, and 7 cervical. The size and shape of each is related to their function. The lumbar are the biggest and strongest of the column with interlocking processes, preventing rotation. This stability is to support the weight of the entire upper body.

Next up is the thoracic. The lower vertabrae are about the same size as the lumbar, but each next, higher vertebrae gets smaller, as each supports less weight. Each thoracic is not as locked in to the next, as the lumbar are, which allows for rotation. We need more general mobility in the thoracic, compared to the lumbar, because this is also where the ribs attach, which have to accommodate breathing.

The top section of the spine, the cervical, has the smallest vertebrae with the least amount of interlock. These only have to support the weight of the head, and require the most mobility (as a unit) of the three regions.

Generally, the overall organization of the bones of the spine is a pyramid: stronger and thicker at the bottom, supporting less weight towards the top. Practically, a pyramid provides stability: a broader base of support with a lower center of gravity means you can stand, walk, or sit with very little muscular effort.

Once you move, however, the pyramid is disrupted, and the muscles have to provide more stability. Let's look at the muscles around the spine, moving from deepest to most superficial.

The deepest layer are the rotatores, each of which connect each vertebrae to the next adjacent, running almost horizontally. Visually, these are stacked from top to bottom, and each individual muscle is very short. Next are the multifidis, which connect each vertebrae diagonally to the next; also stacked top to bottom, and individually not as short as the rotatores. Each individual muscle in these sets of muscles only connects one vertabra to the next. The shortness of these muscles suggests that their function is not so much to twist the spine, as it is to hold the spine steady.

4

The most superficial layers, the semispinalis and the erector spinae, are individually longer, and connect over more than the next vertebrae. Part of the semispinalis connects the head to different points in the thoracic; part of it connects the neck to different parts of the thoracic; and part of it connects the upper portion of the thoracic to the lower portion. Parts of the erector spinae connect the pelvis and thoracic to higher points on the thoracic and cervical spine. These sets of muscles, which can contract over a greater distance, seem more suited to moving the spine (although the functions probably don't break up that neatly).

Compare above the pelvis with below. The pelvis itself is a pretty solid structure of

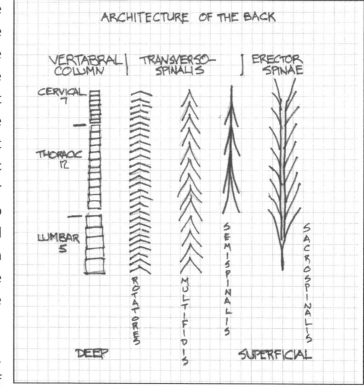

few bones, each significantly bigger than any of the vertebrae. On the back side, a big superficial muscle, the gluteus maximus, connects the pelvis to the femur, and the hamstrings (connect the pelvis to the lower leg. On the front side, part of the quads (rectis femoris) connects the pelvis to the lower leg, while the rest connects the femur to the lower leg.

The system below the pelvis provides for speed and power: big, superficial muscles pull on few, solid beams of bone, moving through large ranges of motion, in few directions. Above the pelvis, there's no muscle match for the glutes or quads; and even if there were, the spine isn't a beam like the femur. With the spine, many muscles only have to hold or move slightly, the next vertebrae. This system provides mobility, with stability, for the overall spine.

What does this suggest about putting a barbell on top of the spine?

With bodyweight alone, the muscles and joints of the spine are fully capable of holding the torso and head steady, while the bigger muscles (glutes, quads, and hams) move the legs and propel the upper body. In this example, the spine does function as a "column". Manual laborers have known this for years: "Lift with your legs, not your back", means "hold your spine steady, while you bend at your hips and knees".

Put a barbell across your shoulders, however, and the situation changes. Now, instead of a decreasing load from pelvis to head, we have dramatically reversed the load: even just a bar at shoulder level is significantly greater than the weight of the head. Neither the muscles nor the vertebrae are structured to support this: the closer the vertebrae are to the head, the smaller they are; and there is no single mass of muscle connecting the lower vertebrae to the head and neck. The same weight that is

5

appropriate to challenge the glutes and quads, working through the largest, strongest bones and muscles in the body, also has to be supported by the dozens of smaller muscles around each individual vertabrae.

Practically, if you squat with a barbell, your back muscles will get stronger, up to a point. But the spine also has discs and nerves that are being loaded with the bar on your back, which doesn't apply to the femur. As the glutes and quads get stronger and need more weight to challenge them, your back is taking on more strain in a variety of ways.

So the idea of working your lower body, by loading a barbell on your shoulders, is limited in several directions. Don't worry; it can get worse: put a barbell on your shoulders and try to exercise one leg at a time.

Balancing on one leg or a split stance relies on small muscles of the hip and deep muscles of the spine.

A fundamental concept in biomechanics is relating your center of gravity to your base of support. You can stand on two feet and maintain your balance pretty much without effort, because your center of gravity falls within your base of support. Pick one foot up, i.e., remove a support, and you should fall to that side, because now, your center is outside your single support.

Generally, though, we don't, by unconsciously shifting our center of gravity away from the foot off the ground, and directly over the foot on the ground. The function of the muscles on the side of the hip (gluteus medius and minimus), in spite of what's implied by hip abduction machines, isn't to pull the femur towards the outside of the pelvis; it's to pull down on the pelvis, shifting the center of gravity towards that side.

It's not a dramatic shift; in fact, it's barely noticeable. If you stand, put your thumbs on the sides of your hip, and pick one foot up to balance on one foot, you can feel the muscle tighten and (if you avoid falling) feel your balance shift. At the same time, the deep muscles around the spine, rotatores and multifidis, tighten, so when the pelvis shifts, the torso follows, maintaining the balance.

The same shift has to happen with exercises. Heel raises, split squats, lunge walking, reverse lunges, stepping up to a bench are all common exercises that disrupt your

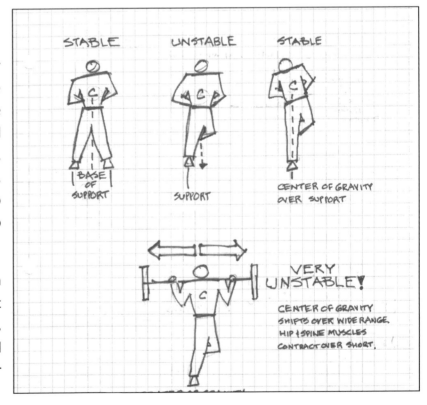

base of support. Your performance of these exercises, conceivably for the prime movers of the lower body, is going to be limited by how well your side hips manage that shift. This is not necessarily a bad thing, because aside from rowing and weightlifting, few sports and physical activities use both legs together as in a leg press or squat. Your inner thigh and outer hip muscles will work extra to stabilize the femur, so the larger muscles can drive the limbs. So you might trade off some intensity for the prime movers, for more stabilization, and in the long run it may even out. The complications start when you try to add resistance.

Using a barbell extends your mass so far to the sides that the normal shift of your center of gravity gets magnified. Instead of your center of gravity being connected to your body mass, it's now connected laterally to the ends of the bar. If the bar isn't placed exactly centered, or if the plates shift at all, or if the wind blows to one side, you don't just have to manipulate your bodyweight; it's your bodyweight, plus the extra moment arms created laterally. If you lose your balance, you're probably better off if the bar falls off than if you try to re-balance, because the spine is going to be unavoidably involved. (Maybe not so good for other people in the gym.)

The safest way to load single-leg or split stance exercises with weight is by keeping the weight close to your center. Weighted vest, one dumbbell on the working side, dumbbells in each hand, weight plate held across the chest, even a hip belt: all these keep the weight closer to your center, and provide similiar work for the lower body stabilizers and prime movers.

Putting the weight back involves much smaller muscles than the ones that lifted it.

You have finished your set without incident. Your muscles might be burning, you're breathing heavier, you have barely locked out the last, most difficult rep. Don't relax yet: you have to maintain lockout until the bar is physically supported by the rack. Your prime movers are shot, so if the weight moves away from zero moment arm, that load is going to have to be supported by much smaller, deeper muscles.

With the squat, if you slouch, relax your gut, or bend forward to put the bar on the stand, the weight moves off center, and the deep muscles of the spine discussed above will try to hold things together. With any amount of weight on your shoulders, this puts the spine in a vulnerable position, so a weight that challenged your glutes and quads is especially dangerous. You have to keep everything tight, walk as short a distance as possible to the rack, position the bar directly over the rack, then set the weight down. Now you can collapse.

The bench press is a bit more complex. Many bench press stations have too much height between the bench and the rack, so you either need a lift off from a partner or you hunch your shoulders forward to get the bar. Bench pressers usually position themselves away from the rack, so it doesn't interfere with the path of the bar; but this means the bar has to move over your forehead, face, jaw, and throat before getting set to press.

This is manageable at the start of the set, but when you're done, you have to reverse everything, and this is where the problems are. At the end of the set, you're locked out: the pecs and triceps are shot, but you can still support the weight. Since the rack is "overhead", you have to move the bar away from directly over your chest, towards the rack. Even though your elbows are still locked, you create a new moment arm, so again, the same weight gets "heavier". Only now, the weight is over your face, and your pecs and triceps are spent.

At the same time, you have to raise the bar to clear the rack. If you lift your shoulders off the bench (protract the scapula), you use the serratus anterior and pectoralis minor. Since both are deeper and smaller than the pectorals, in order for them to move the same weight that exhausted the pectorals, they probably have to heave, not lift under control. The combination of exhausted prime movers, deep muscles trying to move big weight, a new moment arm, and being pinned in place can be a disaster.

A single human spotter may not be much help. Usually the spotter stands centered between the stands, but away from the path of the bar. If the bench presser misses the rack, or gets stuck at the bottom, the spotter has to be able to power clean or deadlift the bar, quickly. I especially like the 200 pound bodybuilder being spotted by the 135 pound partner. Unless that 135 pounder can clean 300 pounds, the best you can hope for is the 911 call.

Ideally, once you finish your set, you stay locked with the weight above your chest, without trying to lift your shoulders or lean the weight towards the rack, while spotters lift the weight to the supports. The minimum setup is to have two, one at each end, to lift and place the bar on the rack, or to hold it off you while you scramble. The best is to have a third, centered, who can steer the bar.

Practical steps to avoid barbell catastrophe

If your tool of choice is the barbell, whether by necessity or preference, you have to take precautions, especially with maximum efforts. You may still get hurt with submax efforts, and you may still get hurt with the precautions in place, but probably not with permanent, life-altering injuries.

Center the bar, and always use collars. Deep muscles make small adjustments for centering and balance. Extending the weight laterally makes excessive demands on them, that will probably never come up in any other context, and is too risky.

Use structural barriers to avoid being pinned by the barbell. Horizontal rails should be sturdy enough and set high enough to keep the bar off you. If you use a smith machine, the bottom stops must be set no lower than the sticking point; don't rely on the hooks.

Use a minimum of 2, preferably 3, human spotters who are paying attention. One at each end of the barbell, to catch and lift it off you, and a center one to steer, either the barbell or you out of the way.

Stay tight at the end of the set. Even with locked knees and elbows, you can still make the weight "heavier" by accidentally creating a new moment arm, which would risk straining the deep muscles and worse. Maintain your posture until the bar is placed in the supports.

To load single-leg or split stance exercises, keep the weight close to you, or use other techniques for progression.   Keeping the extra load close to the center mimics the natural balancing more than the extended weight on a bar. You may choose less risk over more load, and use bodyweight alone, for more reps and sets, and less rest.

Of course, the most direct way to avoid injury with a barbell is: **Don't put a barbell over your spine, face, jaw, and throat.** If you're open to the idea, that is.

For many people, even if the barbell was capable of delivering unique, phenomenal benefits, the risk simply isn't worth it. There are other, effective ways of working the same muscles, and safer, more appropriate ways of loading joints than with the barbell squat and bench press. The barbell is a perfectly adequate tool, especially compared to what was available before it, but it's not magic or super-science.

"Conventional wisdom" has created an aura around certain exercises and approaches that isn't necessarily supported by basic biomechanics. Weights load limbs; deep muscles stabilize joints, so superficial muscles can move the loaded limb; and bones at the joint move in relation to each other. This happens whether you use a barbell, bodyweight, a weight stack, or a rock. There's no magic attached to one technique or tool vs. the other. There are, however, specific, documented ways that muscles and joints are supposed to function, and walking into a gym doesn't change that.

Avoiding catastrophe is really the least you can get out of applying biomechanics to weight training. You can also cut down on unnecessary strain on the joints, and load the muscles more effectively. Fortunately, the two go together.

2. "Full Range of Motion" : Biomechanics or Buzzword?

While it's a lot less prominent now, the phrase "Use a Full Range of Motion" had been an obligatory piece of instruction since the introduction of Nautilus machines in the 1970s. Every magazine article, book, machine instruction card, and fitness person simply had to include it. Although well-intentioned, the concept runs into issues from several directions.

First, the phrase became so overused, that it lost meaning, in that it meant whatever the speaker wanted it to mean. Weight stack equipment implied a certain range of motion; a free weight exercise implied a greater range; an unloaded movement still greater; and a passive range still greater. For example, machine biceps curls with the arms over a pad; standing dumbbell curls; moving your arm from palms down, straight elbow, arm behind you, to palms up, bent elbow, overhead; all involve a different "full range of motion" for the biceps. Exactly which was the important one?

And did it matter? One of the justifications for FROM was to recruit fibers at different joint angles, implying that the fibers that moved a limb part way through a rep were different from the fibers that moved the limb through the rest of the rep, and so by using FROM, all the fibers would be recruited.

Except that a basic concept in muscle science is that fiber recruitment is based on load or speed, not joint angle (for a given muscle). I would footnote this, but it's in the beginning of any textbook on muscle science, and quite a few personal training certification texts.

There's an oddly related concept out there also, which says if you emphasize a particular joint angle, you will get stronger or more developed at that joint angle; which is usually supported by the speakers' observations, and the usual, low-subject-number exercise study, but not entirely by biomechanics.

The Length-Tension Curve

Here is a depiction of a standard graph relating the length of a muscle with the force it produces. This tells us several things that affect Full Range of Motion, angle training, and weight training in general.

11

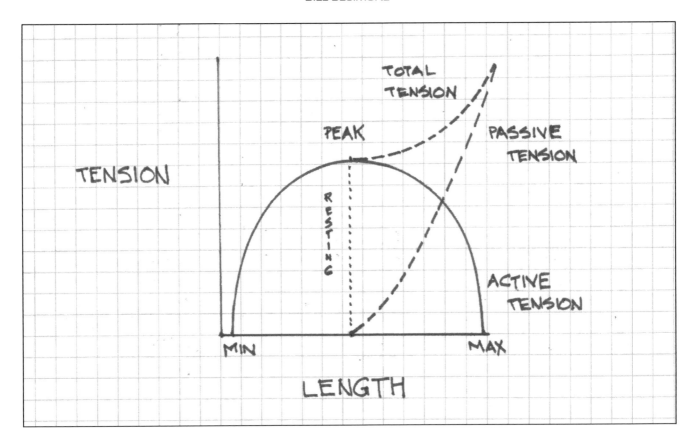

As we voluntarily contract a muscle (on the graph, the "active" line, moving from right to left, or maximum length to minimum length), the muscle gets stronger, then weaker. We're strongest in a range near the middle ("resting" or "favorable" length). We're weakest at the extremes of full contraction and full stretch ("insufficiencies"). But it's not a cliff, it's a slope, so as the muscle length approaches the extremes, strength starts to get affected. In other words, you don't have to be at the extremes for muscle strength to be affected, you just have to approach the extremes.

Generally, in daily life, the body avoids putting the muscles near the weaker positions. But if you insist on using a "full range of motion", or you try to work specific joint angles with isolation exercises (concentration curl, triceps kickbacks, for examples), you will be loading these areas, and all you really do is reduce the weight in your hand. In order to move through the biomechanically weaker ranges, you have to use less weight than if you stayed in the stronger range. Working the weaker ranges won't invert the curve, i.e. make your muscles stronger at the extremes than in the middle, because the curve comes from the most basic muscle science. In practice, no one, for instance, is ever able to use more weight in a concentration curl, than in an upright curl.

Passive Tension And The Full Stretch

If you try to overemphasize the stretch position, other aspects come into play. Notice as you move from Peak Tension to fully stretched, while the "active" curve drops, the Passive and Total Tension curves increase. More load is being supported by the non-contracting parts of the muscle fiber. In daily life, this protects the muscle from a sudden stretch, like when you miss a step or catch something unexpected. But with weights in the stretch position, this (along with the eccentric level of strength) gives the illusion that you're "getting stronger" in that range.

Don't fall for it. If you can lift a weight, you know that you can hold or lower it; but if you're lowering a weight into the stretch, or worse, bouncing into the stretch, you don't really know where your maximum is, until you exceed it. At which point, your first clue might be a ruptured tendon or torn muscle.

Another issue.   When a muscle goes taut, from being overstretched, something else happens: tenodesis, or the tendon action of muscle. Joints will shift to accommodate an overstretched muscle, causing complications at that other joint. The stretched position of a leg curl (flexed hip design) will cause the pelvis to shift, flattening out the lumbar curve. The stretched position of the triceps, during an overhead triceps extension or pullover machine, tries to pull the scapula further forward; but the overhead position has already moved the scapula in that direction, so the muscles that stabilize the scapula may strain. For joints that aren't mobile, you may bring on an acute injury. Dumbbell chest flyes can overstretch the pectorals, and since the sternum doesn't move in that direction, a torn pectoral can result. Old hip adduction designs, that loaded the stretch and didn't limit the range, put a lot of stress on the pubic symphysis, another joint which generally prefers to move only during childbirth.

There might be some metabolic benefit to working in these ranges, but the pattern of muscle force won't change, since it is directly derived from the most fundamental part of muscle science, the sliding filament model. This model describes muscle contraction as overlapping fibers, with the most force resulting not from the beginning of the overlap or complete overlap, but from an optimal overlap somewhere between the two. Unless a training technique undoes the sliding filament model, by rearranging how the actin and myosin overlap at the microscopic level, this pattern of muscle force is what it is, at the level of both the myofibril and intact muscle.

Which begs the question: why use any range of motion at all? If you can't affect the pattern of muscle force, why not just exert effort at the one, peak muscle length?

Because this curve is literally "academic", in that it reflects how a detached muscle behaves. Cut muscle off the bones, stimulate it to contract, load it into a stretch, and this curve is the result. With intact muscles, we have to look at muscle torque curves for a particular joint movement to see where the peaks and slopes are.

Muscle Torque Curves

Muscle torque curves are different for each muscle and joint action, because Length-Tension curve is only one component. Other aspects that go into muscle torque are the internal moment arm and the movement range being tested.

Practically, the force produced by the muscle isn't directly applied to a weight. It's applied to a limb, which pulls or pushes the weight. The internal distance between the tendon and the closest joint creates a lever (or moment arm), which changes as the joint moves. Since muscle torque is the product of muscle force and moment arm (by definition), since both components vary through a movement, the muscle torque also varies through a movement.

Exactly how it varies depends on the muscles, joints, and ranges being tested. The curves for each action differ from each other, and the curves for the same action would differ slightly based on the speed of movement.

Theoretically, if you knew the exact muscle torque curve for a movement, you could design an exercise that varied the mechanical difficulty in exactly the same pattern. This would make the exercise incredibly effective and efficient at using the available muscle force and exhausting the muscle. Isokinetics and cam-based machines tried to do this. Practically, this level of manufactured precision turned out to be a lot harder to effect than it sounds, and it also appears not to be a requirement for a productive workout.

Training the Weak Range?

However, industrial difficulties aside, trying to "bring up" the weak portions of the muscle torque curve, by doing a specific exercise to target the weak range, or overemphasizing that part of the rep, is futile. The variation in muscle torque is mechanical, not malleable. You could only work the weak range for whatever time frame you choose, and you won't be able to significantly change the pattern of muscle torque. Every healthy quadriceps will always show lower muscle torque near full knee extension compared to other knee angles, every healthy biceps will show more muscle torque with the elbow near 90 degrees compared to other angles, and so on. Isolating the weak ranges will bring on more fatigue, and there may be more sensation, but all you are really going to do is reduce the amount of weight in your hand.

You have to be careful that what you identify as a "weak range" is actually the muscle you are trying to work, and not a flaw in the design of the exercise or machine. Circular cams, for instance, don't match muscle torque curves except for a very limited range; so if you can't finish a curl on a machine with a circular cam, it's not that you have a "weak range" in your biceps, the cam is wrong. If you are unable to touch your chest to the bar in a chin up, it's not that your lats are defective; they are expected to be weaker in that position. Trying to touch the chest involves scapular retractors, not the lats, so the design of the instruction ("touch your chest to the bar") is flawed.

It's far more useful to concentrate on training the strong range of the muscle action.

Peak Muscle Torque and the Sticking Point

"Strong range" doesn't mean the point you can handle the most weight. You handle the most weight at lock out, because the weight is supported by the bones and creates zero lever through the joints. This position is next to useless for training purposes, because the bones and connective tissue, not the muscles, bear the load.

The range you should be concerned about is around the joint angle for Peak Muscle Torque. This is the biomechanically strongest position. By matching this position to the most challenging position of the exercise, the exercise design can challenge your muscle strength more effectively and efficiently than loading the weak ranges.

This doesn't require cams and advanced equipment; conventional equipment and free weights, as well as newer devices like the Bodyblade, can be manipulated to do the same thing, which we demonstrate in the Exercises section.

The most challenging position of an exercise is the mechanical sticking point, or a maximum moment arm. With free weights, it is where the weight is at the farthest horizontal distance from the joint ("the end of the seesaw"). With cam-based machines, it's where the chain or cable comes off the largest radius of the cam. With plate-loaded, leverage machines, it is again where the weight is at the greatest horizontal distance from the axis of the loading arm.

For muscle actions where we have a specific muscle torque curve, we matched the sticking point as closely as possible to the joint angle for peak torque.

For those without, the approach was to use an Effective Range of Loading. The general idea was to start with the full range around the joint, and subtract the less useful ranges. Eliminate the lockout (zero moment arm) as it doesn't require muscular effort. Eliminate the extremes of the muscle lengths (the positions of the insufficiencies). Also eliminate any positions of joint obstruction. You're left an exercise that challenges the muscle approximately where it's most capable of applying force, no discernable sticking point or lockout, and less stress on the joints.

"Full range of motion", while a well-intended piece of instruction, was really a product of its time. In the context of bodybuilders doing short pumping motions, and piling on weight for partial lock out reps, it was a step in the right direction. But once it got taken out of context, it went too far in unproductive ways, and created a need for more precise instruction.

Ironically, one reaction to that need was to go the other way, to become deliberately less concerned with specific muscle actions.

3. "Functional Training": Purpose or Practice

It's hard to argue with what appears to be the intent behind functional training. One of the benefits of any exercise program should be to help you deal with the physical demands of your everyday life, and the design of your program should reflect that.

Go back 30 years or so. As the general public became interested in weight training, the only people familiar with weights were bodybuilders, and so everyone tried to train like a bodybuilder. Obviously, unless your goal is bodybuilding, this is completely inappropriate for an athlete, an executive, a homemaker, a physical therapy patient, etc., and so the idea came about of looking at why the person was training, and tailoring the program to the person. In other words, training became more functional, i.e. more related to the intended purpose.

Skip ahead to now. The phrase "Functional Training" has taken over the exercise media, used to justify an incredibly wide range of physical activities. So wide, that the original intent seems lost, and the practice is full of inconsistencies. Is it "working the body as a unit"? Then wouldn't kettlebells and weighted vests become, "a unit, plus". Is it free weight exercises only? Then why do "functional training" catalogs feature pulley and vibration machines? Is it to "prepare you for the demands of daily life"? Wouldn't the things you do in daily life have done that already? Between the serious people doing specific work with their athletes and clients, the personal trainers impressing their clients with their deep knowledge of human tricks, and the catalogs trying to sell affordable equipment rather than multi-thousand dollar machines, the legitimate information gets lost among all the hype and clutter. Let's try to put all these activities in context.

The Good: Moving Limbs vs. Stabilizing Joints

The best parts of "Functional Training" draw a distinction between the muscles that move limbs and the muscles that stabilize joints, and explore appropriate ways of training the stabilizers.

Anyone who weight trains is familiar with the standard, head-to-toe, front-and-back, muscle chart. This isn't a complete inventory; these are the most superficial muscles, the prime movers, the ones that give your physique a shape. Compared to the underlying muscles, these muscles are bigger, have fewer attachments, and are easier to distinguish from each other. Since they're on top, and bigger, they have more internal distance between their angle of pull and the axis of the joint, so they act through a greater internal moment arm. These muscles are most suited for moving limbs and applying torque through the limbs.

Not visible on the standard muscle chart are the deeper layers of muscles, the postural muscles. These have complementary qualities to the superficial muscles. These are smaller or flatter, have many attachments, and often blend with adjacent muscles in anatomy and in function. They are closer to the joints, so they act through much smaller moment arms, and so wouldn't be as suited to move the limbs. The smaller size keeps them out of the way of joint motion, so they are unlikely to grow, or at least grow noticeably; but they still are able to hold the joints together, because muscles are stronger holding or releasing than lifting.

We've already looked at the muscles around the spine. The rotator cuff is an example of separate muscles (supraspinatus, infraspinatus, teres minor, subscapularis) blending with adjacent muscles. The deep muscles around the hip blend in function, with each muscle having different roles in moving or holding the femur, depending on the degree of rotation, flexion, extension, adduction, and abduction. Each joint is similar, in that multiple deeper muscles with different attachments work in different combinations.

Practically, the differences between the postural and prime movers show up in injuries. Rotator cuff problems are more common than deltoid problems; back spasms more common than glute strains. Groin pulls happen, partially because most lower body work (e.g. squat, deadlifts) stabilizes both legs at the same time, so the deep muscles of the hip are relatively untrained.

The interaction between the two sets of muscles is summed up by "you don't fire a cannon out of a canoe". The bigger superficial muscles need a stable platform, provided by the deep muscles holding the joints steady. With that platform, your effort goes directly against the object you're working against, whether it's a barbell, machine, opponent, or the ground. Without that platform, not only is your effort dispersed, the load you push against "pushes back": the deep muscle trying to hold the joint together is now trying to move against that load.

In your workout, your choice between free weights and machines in this regard is almost irrelevant. You should brace your midsection, hold your shoulders down and back, and set your hips and ankles whether you're on a machine, using a barbell, or whatever your tool of choice. It's what you do with your body that counts. You can stabilize your joints on a machine, and you can have poor posture with a free weight; the tool doesn't inherently dictate what happens with the deep muscles.

Training the Core

A more relevant issue is when and how it's appropriate to specifically train the deep muscles. If the rest of your training is done with stable postures, and you seem to get through your daily physical activities without problems, you may be fine without any specific work for the deep muscles. If it's not broke, don't fix it. Conversely, if you've had problems in the past, and if you're not actively injured, a modest amount might be preventive. The key is to not use the same strategies for the deep, as you do for the show muscles.

Remember, the deep muscles are used to holding statically. Holding strength is greater than lifting strength; but another way to look at it is that holding requires less energy than lifting. Simply moving a muscle that is used to holding is more work for that muscle; you don't need to set personal records. This is why, for instance, elastic and light dumbbells are perfectly adequate for rotator cuff work. Concentrate on the movement, not the weight, which will also keep the larger superficial muscles from taking over. For the muscles around the spine, which are used to holding in a vertical posture, simply shifting to horizontal, with planks, bird dogs, side planks, etc. is significantly more load for them to hold.

These aren't your only options; the catalogs are full of them, and some of them may work for you. Before you buy the device, just know what you're trying to accomplish; then disregard the chart of 30 exercises that comes with it and do what you need.

One strategy to be particularly careful of is "Train Movements, Not Muscles". This makes sense when doing specific exercise for the deep muscles. It's almost impossible to isolate the individual deep muscles of the spine, or the hips, or rotator cuff, so using a specific movement (planks, birddog; one leg balance; Bodyblade) for the general area works. It makes less sense if you're combining Big Muscle Movements: squats with curls, walking lunges with presses, wood choppers and squats. The work for the bigger muscles is going to be limited by the smaller muscles, but more importantly, the weights are going to be constantly throwing your center of gravity off. Are you concentrating on your leg movements, your arm movements, or managing your postures? To me, the cost of mismanaging your spine posture is far too high for whatever benefits are touted. If you really feel the need to train "movements" in this way, my suggestion is to use other ways of adding challenge than using weights: stricter form, slower movements, less rest between sets.

Of course, practicing the actual techniques in a sport, martial art, dance, etc. is real "training movements". If you really feel the need to "do something more athletic", I suggest you do an actual real-world activity, not mash together weight training movements.

The combination movements are hard work, however. Your breathing gets heavy, your muscles burn, you may get nauseous, all very compelling; but this leads to the real concern about "Functional Training".

And, the Not So Good

The worst parts of "Functional Training" blur the distinctions between the muscles that move limbs and the muscles that stabilize joints, and risk long-term joint health for the sake of today's "hard workout".

The barbell squat, for instance, is generally considered a more functional exercise than the leg press. You'll get no argument from me that a hard set of barbell squats is, overall, more physically draining than a hard set of leg presses. And the barbell squat certainly requires more balance and knowing where your body is in space (proprioception) than the leg press. Yet, when you look at the bones and muscles above the pelvis compared to below, the leg press does appear to load the body more appropriately (as detailed previously). And when you look at the body's mechanisms for balance and proprioception, a barbell is a curious choice to address those. Regarding the barbell squat as "Functional" emphasizes today's hard workout over concerns for the long term health of the spine.

Rotating and bending are also considered "Functional", in that they're usually categorized as part of people's daily activities. Up and down "woodchops" using pulleys or elastic, medicine balls, kettlebells are all used to train rotation. The problem is that in practice, there is a slight difference between a "turn" and a "twist", but there's a huge difference in effect on the spine. With a turn, the hips and shoulders stay in the same plane, held there by the muscles around the spine and midsection. This movement is worth practicing, under control, so that when you actually do it in real life (lifting a load out of a car trunk, swinging a baseball bat, golf club, etc.) your body has done it before and knows how to do it. Sports coaches teach it all the time: "Get your hips into it".

Same thing with bending: "Bend from the hips" or "Lift with your legs, not your back" refers to hip hinging. You hold your spine steady, with the normal curves, and bend at the hips and knees. The muscles around your spine maintain the spine posture, while the bigger muscles of the hips and thighs provide the force and motion.

The potential problems start when, from either fatigue or losing focus, the turns and hip hinges turn into twisting and bending the spine. The first risk is to the deep muscles, which may strain and go into spasm, but the more important and long term risk is to the disc. The normal curves in the back keep the load on the discs even. While the spinal column curves, the discs stay flat. Flatten a curve in the spine, or bend it more, and one side of the disc gets pinched while the other pushes out. Twist the spine, and the top half of the disc moves with the top vertebrae, while the bottom stays in place or goes opposite; like wringing out a wet towel. You can do this one time, a handful of times, maybe even years of times, and get away with it; but repeated over time, and neither situation is good for the long term health of the disc.

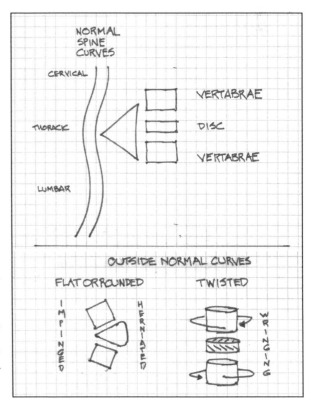

A Safer Approach

If you are using rotation and bending movements in your workout, check yourself. Are you concentrating on turning and hip hinging, or is muscle burn and heavy breathing distracting you? If you are using combination movements, (dumbbell row while lunging, curls while squatting, etc.), are you paying attention to your trunk, or are you just getting through the set and hoping for the best? Group workouts, kettlebell classes, boot camps, infomercial circuit-style training all use these movements, and they're all hard work, but you may be focused on the effort and not paying attention to your spine. Even if you avoid an immediate injury, even if you do lose bodyfat and get stronger, joint wear-and-tear from the exercise itself doesn't get erased. It accumulates. People who don't exercise, and bend and twist any number of times in daily life, end up with herniated discs and other back problems. Do this deliberately, or inadvertently, in your workouts, and not only are your reps and sets adding to your count of daily life bends and twists, you may be adding speed and resistance to it. "I've done this for years and haven't had any problems"... yet. Past performance is no guarantee of future results.

If your daily life requires you to use bad body mechanics, fix the bad body mechanics in the first place, don't practice them in your workout. Adding reps, speed, and weight to bad body mechanics will just accelerate the wear-and-tear, not make you invulnerable.

Carry loads close to your body. Put the heavy weight plates on trees at chest level. Turn, don't twist. Lift with your legs, not your back. Learn technical instruction in sports, and ergonomics at work.

Then in your workout: Train the superficial muscles with your tool of choice. Consciously stabilize your posture while doing so. If you need to train deeper muscles separately, use light weights, elastics, the appropriate devices (vibration plates, Bodyblades, etc.), or reposition your bodyweight. Save the heavy metabolic challenge for exercises and activities that don't put the spine in a vulnerable position.

Consider avoiding exercises that draw a fine line between "safe" and "dangerous" and don't allow room for fatigue or distraction. But if you simply must do them, do them when you're fresh and can focus on perfect form. It doesn't help if your training is "functional", and you're not.

4. Shaping Muscle or Straining Joints

Open any fitness or muscle magazine, and you're bound to find instructions on changing how your muscles look. Not just in the general sense of losing the fat around the waistline and over the muscles, and building or toning what was under the fat, but in the very precise sense of shaping specific aspects of muscles. Concentration curls are claimed to peak the biceps, while curls over a stand claim the lower biceps. Knee extensions are claimed to develop the lower heads of the quads. Shoulder presses with the bar in front are claimed to develop the front of the shoulder, while presses behind the head, the side of the shoulder. Pullovers are claimed to strengthen the lats in the stretch position; pulling the hands past the chest on rows and chins, the peak position.   Triceps pressdowns are claimed to develop the lateral head, and kickbacks the medial head. Or vice versa.

Once you've picked an exercise, then you're offered a number of tweaks to further refine your sculpting.   Changing your foot positions during squats and leg presses supposedly develop separate parts of the thigh; same with calves. Chins and pulldowns with the elbows parallel supposedly develop different parts of the lats than with the elbows wide. Dips supposedly develop all three heads of the triceps, unless you're bent forward, in which case they develop the chest. We're advised to keep our elbows in during triceps exercises, or other muscles do the work. And so on.

For any exercise, you'll find claims that if you do partial reps in a very specific portion of the rep, you'll either develop more strength in that range or develop the portion of muscle that you feel at that joint angle.

Muscle Isolation, and Does It Matter?

As usual, there is a hint of truth in these claims. In recent years, EMG studies have been published which show more activity in specific heads of muscle compared other heads of the same muscle, depending on the exercise. What the studies don't establish, is if that means anything. If I do an exercise that lights up only the lateral head of the triceps, and do no other triceps exercise, does that mean the lateral head will overdevelop compared to the rest of the triceps? The studies don't establish that. The immediate effect of using an exercise which isolates one head of a muscle, compared to one that uses more of the muscle, is that you use less weight in the isolated exercise; but whether that results in a visually or functionally different muscle over time is unclear. It's asserted that it happens, but it's not addressed in the studies.

Visually, compare physiques. Take, for example, bodybuilders in the Arnold era (late '70s), or fitness models today. Each physique retains a distinctive look, even though they apparently use many of the same exercises, techniques, (and probably ergogenic aids). If shaping in this way was possible, the physiques of everyone using the same exercises should end up looking the same; which is clearly not the case. If two people use the exact same exercise for an extended time, if their muscles had different shape to start, at the end, their muscles will still have different shapes. If one person uses one exercise for an extended time, then switches exercises for an extended time, or if that person uses a different exercise on the right side compared to the left, the muscle shape will also stay the same.

(The one definite way to change the shape of your muscles is to forget tweaking the exercises and do as I did: rupture the biceps and triceps on the same arm. Now, *that* changes the look of your arms.)

"Feeling" the Muscle Work

Prior to the EMG studies, however, the most compelling argument for the shaping strategy was sensation, i.e. "feel". Sure enough, when you did the exercises as prescribed, you would feel the peak of the biceps or the teardrop by the knee or get sore in a different area. These tweaks do create a different sensation in the working muscles and joints. So that must mean it's working, right?

Why? Why associate that "feel" with physiology or biomechanics? I don't know why, either, other than in the absence of any other explanation, it was the only one available. Now, though, better information is handy.

There are several reasons why you would "feel" an exercise differently, none of which having to do with "shaping" the muscle or strengthening a specific joint angle. Keep in mind, that the bigger, superficial muscle is only one component of how your limbs move: the stabilizing muscles, and the shape of the bones at the joint also influence their path.

- You are trying to use the deeper, postural muscles to move a load intended for the larger, superficial muscles (substitution).
- You are working in the weak range of the length-tension curve.
- You are trying to move the limbs, under load, outside of the natural path of the joint.

Substitution

One way to "feel" an exercise is to "squeeze" the finish of the repetition. The superficial muscles have moved the limbs into the finish position of the exercise, and before returning the weight to begin the next rep, you try to get a bit more effort out of the big muscles by squeezing.

In several exercises, though, that last squeeze involves the deeper postural muscles trying to move the same weight. For chest exercises, raising your shoulders off the bench in a bench press, touching the pads of a pec dec together, rolling your shoulders forward on a cable flye are all examples of protraction of the scapula, which is not a function of the pectorals, but of the serratus on the side of the ribcage. The serratus is important in raising the arm overhead, as part of scapulo-humeral rhythm, but trying to move bench press levels of weight is likely to strain it.

For chin ups and pulldowns, "touching your chest to the bar" creates a tightening sensation. Your lats have done their job in bringing your arms next to your ribcage (shoulder extension); the extra squeeze is actually retraction of the scapula, by the trapezius, rhomboids, and other deep muscles of the back. Keeping your shoulders away from your ears during the pull has already engaged these muscles; the squeeze means your performance in the pull will be limited by fatigue in these muscles, not your lats.

In heel raises, "stand on tiptoe at the top of the rep" engages the deep muscles of the feet, as the main role of the calves is to lift the heel or point the foot. Standing on tiptoe is done by making a bow (as in bow and arrow) of the bottom of the foot.

Various exercises for the "glutes" involve short ranges at the end of hip motion (abduction during bodyweight, machine, or cable abduction). The "burning" during these movements isn't from shaping the biggest muscle in the area. It is from using the deeper hip muscles (gluteus medius, minimus, and others), whose role is primarily stability for the pelvis and hip joint, to try to lift weights.

In general, any time you overemphasize the finish position of a rep, you may be switching effort from the prime mover to a deeper muscle, which may not be able to handle the load, and certainly won't benefit the prime mover. Even if you don't substitute, though, the finish position is not necessarily the most important part of the rep.

Working In A Weak Range Of The Muscle Torque Curve

Every muscle provides a varying level of strength (muscle torque), resulting in a range of Peak Muscle Torque; i.e. a range where the muscle is biomechanically strongest. Every exercise has a sticking point, a maximum moment arm; i.e. a point where the exercise is mechanically hardest.

For exercises that mismatch these two aspects, you feel a very distinct strain at the position of maximum moment arm. Examples are triceps kickbacks, dumbbell raises, dumbbell pullovers, bench back extensions. Other exercises position the muscle at the extremes of its length, so the moment arm is irrelevant; the muscle work is limited by its weakest ranges. Examples of this are crunches, sissy squats, concentration curls, wrist curls, and machine leg extensions and curls.

For exercises that are congruent, i.e. exercises where the joint angle for peak muscle torque matches the maximum moment arm, the only "feel" is of overall effort. You don't feel one particular joint angle or aspect of the muscle.

How you perform congruent exercises influences their "feel". If you lockout, you may notice distinct sticking points, because you move from zero moment arms (and so, no effort required) through maximum moment arms (high effort required). But if you don't lock out, your effort feels more even through the rep. Non-lock squats, leg presses, chest presses, chins, pulldowns, curls (coincidentally, the basics) all lack a point of "feel", unlike the "shaping" exercises, but they are all more efficient as using your effort, and allow you to use comparatively more weight.

We'll look at specific muscles and exercises in the "User's Guide". One general point, though, is that it's less important to find a perfect match, than it is to avoid the obvious mismatches. As long as you avoid loading the extreme stretch or contracted positions, you have a margin of error. The exact joint angle for peak torque changes with changes in speed, so the best we can do is approximate. Your body will make the minor adjustments to compensate, so you can address the more obvious concerns.

One of those concerns that should be obvious, but hasn't been, is whether you are performing safe joint motions in the first place.

Moving Outside The Natural Path

Just because you can move a limb a certain way, doesn't mean you should, and it certainly doesn't mean you should move it that way with extra weight. Each joint has unique concerns, so you should study each separately, but a few cover a variety of general exercise movements. Let's start with the shoulders, and moving your arms overhead.

Without a weight in your hand, lift your arm overhead. You probably moved somewhere in the "three quarter" plane (10 or 2 o'clock), because this is the least obstructed path. To demonstrate one obstruction, lift your arms parallel to each other, with your palms up (pure shoulder flexion, full supination of the wrist, external rotation of the shoulder). Notice that at about shoulder level, you are limited from moving further overhead by a tightness in the shoulders. To give the illusion of moving further up, there are several adjustments you could make: you'll arch your back, or lift your ribcage, or lean to one side, or shrug your shoulders. But if you try to move directly overhead, without those compensations, the ligaments in your shoulder twist and bind when your arms reach shoulder height. To actually move your arm higher, you have to fold your arms in (internally rotate), which relieves the binding.

A number of exercises force you either into this "binding" position, or the compensating position. For pulldowns or chin ups with a straight bar (palms up, grip at shoulder width or closer) as your upper arms move above the shoulder, your elbows tend to flare out in order to affect the internal rotation to relieve the strain. Old pullover machines (from various manufacturers) placed pads against the elbow and provided a bar to grip, so shoulders couldn't rotate; instead, you lifted your ribcage and arched your spine, in order to reach the "overhead" stretch. Free weight pullovers with a straight bar or single dumbbell, and overhead triceps exercises also need the shoulders to rotate as your arms and the weight move towards the stretch. The sensation in the shoulders as we tried to "maintain strict form" had nothing to do with improving the strength, shape, function of our lats, triceps, or any other muscle, and everything to do with stressing the ligaments in this position.

And to add insult to injury, the joint angles for peak torque for those muscles aren't near the overhead position. Peak muscle torque for shoulder extension (pulldowns and chin ups) is where your upper arms are at shoulder height (90 degrees of shoulder flexion). For the triceps, when the elbow is overhead and bent, it is stretched over two joints (elbow and shoulder), and so it is at its weakest length.

The other obstruction is straight to the side. With your arm by your side, palm facing back, elbow pointed directly to the side, try to move overhead, as if you had your back against a wall and your arm had to stay in contact with the wall (abduction with internal rotation). Again, about 90 degrees, you meet a bony obstruction; turn your arm so your palm faces front, and you can continue overhead easily. Don't rotate your arm, and you will impinge muscle, ligaments, and other soft tissue between your upper arm and collarbone, leading over time, to a number of joint issues.

The upright row with a barbell puts you into this obstruction, as can dumbbell side raises if you "pour water" (turn the pinky up, as the magazines advised). Machine designs are inconsistent; some position you (correctly) in external rotation, others drive you right into the obstruction. Decline chest exercises, especially with dumbbells or an extreme range of motion also put you in the obstruction.

Using momentum to ignore these obstructions doesn't erase the strain; it just happens to quickly for you to notice. Bouncing out of the bottom on a chin up, quickly pulling a kettlebell into an upright row, bouncing out of the bottom with dips still adds to the wear-and-tear. Yet, of course, these exercises "feel" like they're doing something.

The wrist also affects multiple exercises. The issue here is how a straight bar interacts with the wrist joint. When you use a "palm down" grip (pronated, as in a bench press, press, variations of pulldowns and chins, rows, etc.) it appears that the wrist pivots 180 degrees. Actually, the hand makes the full rotation, because the hand has many more bones, muscles, and joints than the wrist. The "wrist" is limited, because one bone in the forearm (the radius, thumb-side) crosses over the other (ulna, pinky-side) and so is blocked from twisting fully. The wrist only appears to fully pronate by the elbow flaring out and the hand continuing to twist.

This doesn't affect a conventional barbell bench press, because generally, the elbows move away from the sides. It does affect reverse curls, reverse wrist curls, and especially triceps exercises. Conventional instruction has advised us to "keep the elbows in" as a way of focusing the exercise; again, more strain, misinterpreted as benefit.

One last prominent joint to look at is the knee. Machine instruction implies that the knee is a hinge ("line up your knee with the axis of the machine"). Technically, the knee slides-and-rolls, so it's not a pure hinge. The axis moves when the knee bends or straightens, so you actually can't line up your knee with one axis. But for most of the leg extension or leg curl, it functions similiarly to a hinge.

The ends of the motions, however, are different. When you lock out the knee, terminal rotation occurs: an involuntary twisting of the lower leg onto the femur, caused by the shape of the bones, the locking or screw-home mechanism. This allows you to stand or walk with minimal muscular effort. This also means that squeezing the last few degrees at the top of the leg extension, which takes a lot of muscular effort, is a waste of muscular effort.

If your foot is free to move, when you straighten your knee all the way, the shin rotates laterally (to the side). If your foot is planted, the thigh would rotate medially (towards the center). In the knee extension machine, your lower legs are pushing against a movement arm, and you sit on your thighs. The shin and thigh can't move freely to accommodate the terminal rotation, but rotation still has to occur. There will be some rolling of the thighs or shins against the pads, not because the trainee is undisciplined, but because this is how the bones fit. This extra movement (the rolling) is actually a good marker for where to end the rep, because the actual rotation is internal and may not be visible. If you insist on the last few degrees, you are taking a bony lock that is supposed to passively support bodyweight, applying an external load to it, and applying internal effort to force it into place. Your quads will burn, but again, more unnecessary joint stress in order to "feel" the exercise. And also again, far from the joint angle for peak muscle torque for the quads.

Incidentally, you're also working against your knee if you try to squat or leg press, and direct your thighs in an extreme direction. Trying to keep the thighs parallel through the rep, or forcing the knees apart to affect more adduction, also isn't natural. When the knee flexes, if the foot is free, it moves towards the center line, again, due to the shape of the bones in the knee joint. If the foot is planted, when the knee bends, the knee has to move away from the center. Forcing the thighs either straight ahead or directly to the side doesn't allow the knee to do either, creating some knee strain, and has more effect on the deep muscles of the hip and groin trying to stabilize in this awkward position than on the quads or hamstrings.

As compelling as it is, "feel" just isn't that significant in getting any kind of actual result from exercise. The whole idea of shaping and sculpting and selectively tweaking the results you get from your workout might be romantic, but unfortunately, there's also a grounded explanation. The real issue with doing multiple exercises, and multiple versions of exercises, isn't just the questionable benefit to the muscle, but the extra, unnecessary wear-and-tear that comes with it. In the next section, we'll explore why minimizing that is so important.

5. Strength, Speed, and the Human Machine

For all the muscle media devoted to how to lift weights, do we ever ask: Should we lift weights in the first place? The health benefits of exercise are well-documented and widely touted, but most of the benefits are attached to any regular exercise, not just weight training. Consider this:

"Most of the skeletal muscles operate at a considerable mechanical disadvantage. Thus, during sports and other physical activities, forces in the muscles and tendons are much higher than those exerted by the hands or feet on external objects or the ground."

In other words, whatever you do- punch, throw, hit, kick, run, lift a barbell, swing a kettlebell, push a machine- the internal forces placed on your joints are dramatically higher than the external result. Not only does that sound inefficient, it can't be good for your joints.

It happens to be true, by the way, although not entirely a deal-breaker. Before we look at how and why that is, any guesses where this came from? A physical therapist? Chiropractor? Orthopedic surgeon? Yoga instructor? Pilates instructor? Exercise police? Achy, 50-something trainers?

No. It came from the textbook for the personal training certification for the National Strength and Conditioning Association. Which is incredibly ironic, considering that many of the activities featured by the NSCA (Olympic lifts, plyometrics, running drills, etc.) use ballistic movements and momentum, and require a lot of technique to perform correctly. Combine that with, as their own text points out, the inherently high internal forces, and you are left with little margin for error.

The explanation starts in the levers. Most personal training and biomechanics texts go into extensive detail on first, second, and third class levers; axes, fulcrums, moment arms, torque; calculating mechanical advantage; laws of the lever; and so on. And while all that might (?) be interesting, in the gym, it's more useful conceptually than specifically.

All you need to know about the internal forces can be demonstrated with a walnut and a nutcracker.

27

Busting Nuts

Take an ordinary walnut in your hand, and try to crack the shell with your grip alone. No smashing it on a table, simply squeeze your fist around the walnut. Of course, it's far too hard: a lot of effort and discomfort in the hand without result, which is why Man invented Tools.

With the nutcracker, you place the walnut close to the joint, and you apply your grip as far away as you can.   What happens? With a fraction of the effort of the bare-handed attempt, you easily crack the shell. Did you get stronger? Did the shell get weaker? No, but you did use "leverage": the distance between the joint and the resistance (the walnut) is much shorter than the distance between the joint and the effort (your grip). This kind of tool "leverages" force: a little effort away from the joint creates a greater force close to the joint. A crowbar, a wheelbarrow, a car jack all work off the same principle.

What you would never do is to grip the nutcracker close to the joint, and place the walnut at the ends. You could try, and you'll have nearly the same result as trying barehanded: much effort and discomfort in your hands, and not enough force the crack the nut.

Applying effort close to a joint is ineffective at amplifying force, in fact, it reduces the usable force; but it is very effective at amplifying distance. It's still a valid lever; it's just used for different purposes. Tweezers, barbecue tongs, baseball bats, hockey sticks, golf clubs, all move a greater distance at the far end of the tool, than where the effort is applied.   Any movement near the joint creates greater movement at the ends.

Levers, in general, then, can be one of two types: they either amplify force, or they amplify distance; and they have opposite traits. If they amplify force, a little effort in, creates great effort out, although that effort is applied over a very short distance. If they amplify distance, a little movement applied near the joint, creates a greater movement at the far end, although that movement at the far end is not very forceful. And it is "either/or"; the same device can't leverage both force and distance at the same time. (This analysis, by the way, comes from outside the exercise literature, from Steven Vogel, **Cat's Paws and Catapults** and **Prime Mover.**)

Where do the human muscles and joints (at least, the superficial ones) fall in these categories?

Limbs and Levers

Look at your elbow where the biceps attaches. Move the closest part of your forearm an inch; how far does your hand move? Now the shoulder: move your arm in the "side raise" motion, so that the edge of your deltoid moves an inch. How far does your hand move? A little movement at the joints creates a much larger movement at the ends of the limbs. Human limbs, like fly swatters, tweezers, etc., amplify distance.

And like all distance amplifiers, the effort that goes into the shorter movement near the joint, is reduced at the moving end of the lever. Or, as in the earlier quote, "...forces in the muscles and tendons are much higher than those exerted by the hands or feet..." The human skeleton is inherently built to leverage distance, not force. A little movement goes into the joint, much movement comes out. Great force goes into the joint, less force comes out.

The good thing about leveraging distance is that it also leverages speed. Since it takes the same time for short movement near the joint, as it does for the longer movement near the end, the end is moving faster: it covers greater distance over the same time. A fly swatter works this way. Ordinarily, a fly is too fast to catch by hand; but the end of the fly swatter covers more distance than your hand, in the same time, so it amplifies your hand speed. With your limbs, the foot moves a greater distance than your hip in the same time; your hand moves a greater distance than your shoulder in the same time; and so on.

As a force producer, however, the human skeleton is inefficient, since greater force goes into the joint than comes out at the hand or foot. To demonstrate: hold a yardstick horizontally, with each hand at the end of the yardstick. Now slide one hand towards the other, so that one hand is holding one end, and the other is at the one-inch mark. Which position puts more pressure at the "joint"? Even though you hold the same amount of weight (you are holding the same yardstick), the close position obviously puts more pressure on your fingers. The same analysis applies to our limbs and muscles. The yardstick represents our limbs, and our fingertips represent where our muscles attach to the limbs (close to the joint).

To our interest, for safe joint function during exercise, the effort that goes in, that gets reduced at the ends of the limbs, is being absorbed by the bones, tendons, and soft tissue that make up the joint, not by the object at the foot or hand. This may not be an immediate concern, or even cause an acute injury, but over time, it accumulates, and may show up as irritation, inflammation, tendinitis, bursitis, and so on. Even if your exercise form was perfect, exercise does tend to be progressive, so you always add to this; and of course, the normal wear-and-tear of daily life counts, too.

From the levers, alone, it would appear that the human machine is built for speed, not strength.

Speed, Force, and Power

In real life activities, however, the speed advantage of the skeleton isn't separate from the force production; the two aspects interact, as in the graph below.

The graph refers to how a given muscle performs at different speeds. On the left, we have zero speed: isometric, or a static contraction; no movement occurring. On the right, maximum speed, movement as fast as possible. The force curve moves in a downward slope from left to right. At zero speed, you generate the most force, as compared to faster speeds; which is consistent with the conventional wisdom of isometric strength being greater than positive strength. The curve is also consistent with muscle torque curves at different speeds, which show faster speeds resulting in lower muscle torque; leading to a minimum force at the fastest speed.

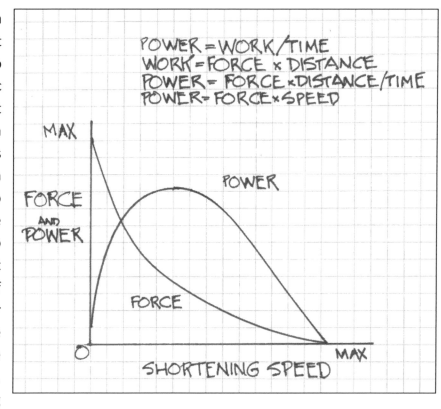

What this graph tells us about Force is not new; but what is significant is what it tells about Power. Power doesn't come from Speed alone or Force alone, but is the product of the two. By definitions:

- Power = Work / Time
- Work= Force X Distance
- Power= Force X Distance/Time
- Distance/Time=Speed
- Power=Force X Speed

On the graph, where Force is at its' maximum (at zero speed), Power is at a minimum. Where Speed is at a maximum, Force is at zero; Power is again at a minimum. Unlike Speed or Force, which each peak at an extreme, Power peaks at an optimal combination of the Speed and Force.

With regard to physical performance, this suggests that the right combination works better than either extreme; unless, of course, the competition is specifically for one of the extremes. This is where practicing technique for sports, martial arts, dance, or any physical activity comes into play. In addition to whatever other benefits the practice offers, it keeps you from relying on brute force or speed, so that you find the optimal combination for power.

The graph applies, however, to how a given muscle reacts at a moment in time. Improve the overall strength of the muscle, and the overall Power curve would shift up. Still zero at the extremes, but the peak would be higher, and the slopes would become progressively higher, if that given muscle became capable of exerting more overall force.

So Do We Train With Weights Or Not?

Wait a second, you're thinking, you're contradicting yourself.

I just explained how the human levers are designed to leverage speed, not force, and that the wasted force gets absorbed by the joints, leading to theoretical problems down the road. This might suggest avoiding weight training.

But then I present information that in the physical world, Power unavoidably involves Force. And since weight training can improve overall muscle force, this suggests including weight training. So which is it?

Well, both sets of conditions are opposing, and true. The inherent nature of the musculoskeletal lever puts high internal forces on the joints; and physical performance (power) can be improved with improved muscle force. Joint wear-and-tear is cumulative, and health benefits come with regular exercise.

The answer is to train with weights, just in a way that acknowledges the risk of future problems. And hopefully, avoids it, although joint wear is cumulative from everything you do in life, not just exercise. Bad posture, bad body mechanics at work, bad form in sports, bumps and bruises also work against you, but the idea is to not add to it, more than necessary, with your exercise.

And specifically, by your exercise selection. If you've avoided the tragic accident, and if you've moderated the range of motion, and if you're utilizing the best of "functional training" and avoiding the worst, and if you've given up on "shaping" your muscles, the next step is to match proper muscle and joint function with specific exercises to do in the gym. Given the nature of the levers, and the cumulative aspects of joint wear, these exercises aren't a guarantee against joint problems, but they are intended to not make things worse while still being effective at training muscle. In the next section, we'll look at specific exercises you can do with commercial equipment and in a home gym, and more importantly at the appropriate joint positions and movements.

6. Congruent Exercises: A User's Guide

These exercises are designed to be congruent in two ways: first, to protect the joints, and second, to efficiently challenge the muscles.

Range of Loading

The photos show the start and finish limb position of each exercise: the "effective range of loading". We already discussed how the nature of the musculoskeletal levers places disproportionate forces on the joint. By designing the exercises to avoid bony locks, ligament binding, and bony obstructions, we minimize unnecessary strain on the joints and the deep muscles.

At the same time, the demonstrated ranges pretty closely match the changes in muscle torque to changes in resistance torque. Where you are biomechanically strong, the exercise is mechanically difficult; and where you are biomechanically weaker, the exercise is mechanically easier. The sensation is just one of effort throughout the range. This is more efficient at using your muscular effort, compared to an exercise with a distinct sticking point and lock-out.

As a regular practice, try not to exceed the "ranges of loading" as shown, whether on these exercises or alternatives. If you do, you probably won't suffer an immediate injury; but, as a habit, you don't want to add wear-and-tear. Some machine designs don't allow you to set a specific range, and so you have to move through a poor joint position. Doing that twice in a set—before the first rep, and after the last—is better than doing so on every rep. Or, if you're particularly motivated, you may want to lock out to gather yourself, to get that "extra" rep. Again, as a regular practice, there are safer ways to accomplish the same, but occasionally may not hurt.

33

With regard to alternative exercises: the brand name on the machine, or the jargon for an exercise, is much less important than what your joints and muscles do. So if your gym has a different brand of equipment, or if you only have barbells or prefer bodyweight, you can always keep the specific joint concerns in mind and adjust as best you can.

Exercise Form and Posture

You should do the exercises with as little momentum, either way, as possible: don't heave the weight up or drop the weight back. Steady pressure, a brief pause, and a steady, controlled release to another pause. Done this way, most of these exercises "will just feel hard"; there won't be a sticking point or a dead spot.

While you're doing this, you should have as little movement as possible from the rest of your body. Don't look around, kick your feet, shrug, wiggle, arch your back, etc. On the other hand, the rest of your body shouldn't be completely slack, either. The appropriate strategy is to brace the rest of your body (a moderate static contraction), so the moving limb doesn't also move your pelvis, spine, or shoulder girdle. Muscle contraction works both ways, on the moving limb and on the torso or pelvis; as does the external resistance. Not only do the prime movers work more efficiently against a stable platform, but if that platform shifts, the deep muscles around the joint and the soft tissue have to bear the load. You may focus on straightening the elbow during a chest press, but the resistance is pushing through your shoulder girdle, so the rotator cuff and muscles around the shoulder blades have to stabilize. You may focus on straightening the knee during lower body exercises, but the resistance loads through your pelvis, which directly affects your lumbar spine. The safest approach is to actively stabilize your trunk and limbs; not so much that you move the uninvolved limbs to cheat, but enough to provide the stable platform.

Specifically, you should:

- Hold your shoulder blades down and back;
- Don't exaggerate your neck position;
- Keep a lumbar curve (don't exaggerate a pelvic tilt);
- Maintain a soft lock at the knee (standing exercises);
- Center the weight on your feet (standing).

With these lower body exercises, the goal is to challenge the muscles while avoiding the disc and deep muscle strain that comes with loading the spine in compression and in flexion. You would also like to protect the knees. You may not get the same feel of overall effort with these, compared to barbell squats and dead lifts. Your effort will be more localized to the actual muscles you're trying to work, and not towards keeping your spine and rib cage from collapsing.

With these upper body exercises, the goal is to challenge the muscles without straining the rotator cuff, the discs and deep muscles of the upper portions of the spine, or the muscles that control the scapula. You would also like to protect the elbows. You may lose the feeling of overall effort that comes with high effort combined with sloppy form, and you'll also lose the alleged shaping sensation. But, your effort will go towards actual muscle work without unintended joint consequences.

HIP-BELT SQUAT

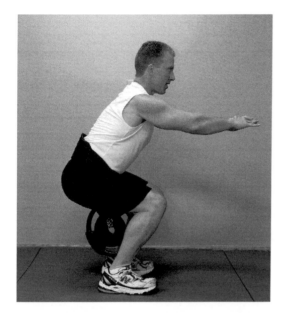

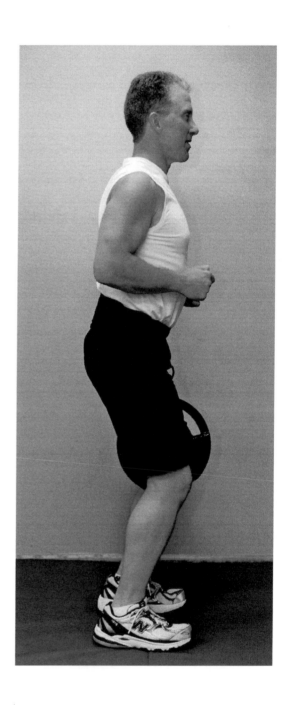

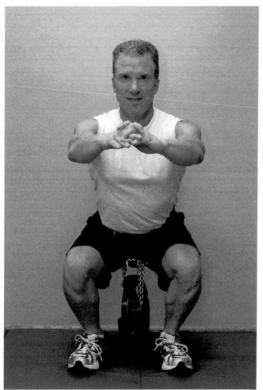

Start position:
A. Arms forward
B. Knees apart

Finish position
A. Arms By sides
B. Knees unlocked

If you can manage the practical aspects of getting in and out of a weighted belt, this is simply the most congruent lower body exercise conceivable: absolutely no compression of the discs; the deep muscles around the spine maintain the posture of the spine as you lean forward; the weight loads through the pelvis; and the natural moment arms adequately match resistance and muscle torque changes. You also would start at the bottom position, so no nasty surprises would come from overloading a standing start. There are some practical concerns, however, that require some work-arounds.

You have to manage your center of gravity differently with the resistance under your hips. As you lower into a squat with a bar on the shoulders, the weight forces you to lean forward. With the weight under your hips, you have to actively lean forward as you squat, or you'll fall back. Depending on your proportions, you may have to project your arms forward at the bottom to balance.

You also have to prepare for the last rep, so you don't drop the plates on your feet, or collapse and land on the plates between your legs. Unfortunately, there's no graceful way out of the belt, especially when your legs are shot and you use a significant amount of weight. Adjust the belt so the plates barely clear the floor at the bottom position, so you don't have too far to get the weight to the floor. Years ago, Nautilus and other manufacturers made platforms for belt squats, which provided some structure for an easier exit. Absent that, you might be better off with especially slow repetitions, not locking out, and longer sets, to make a lighter weight feel heavier. Save the heavy weights for when you have access to the next exercise.

- **Match your spine curves to the curves in the seat**

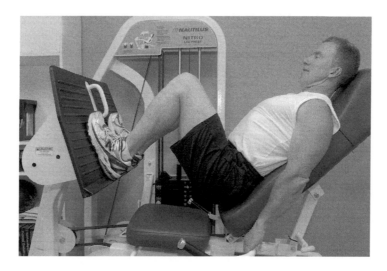

- **Allow some space between the calves and hamstrings, and between thighs and torso, at the start position (shown)**

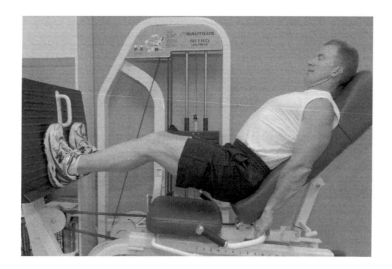

- **Knees unlocked at the finish**

The model shown has the curves built into the seat back that follow the curves of the spine. Unfortunately, it doesn't provide a way of elevating the seat, so depending on the height of the user, the curves may not align. Either use pads on the seat bottom, or align the back and leave space between the seat and the user. The seat angle should be set as low as possible to mimic the torso angle of a free-hand squat. If the seat is too vertical, in addition to flattening the lumbar curve at the bottom, your legs approach lock-out short of the joint angle for peak muscle torque for the glutes. Leave some space between the calves and the hamstrings at the start position to avoid the crow-bar effect on the knee.

SPLIT SQUAT

Start position:
- **Back heel up**
- **Effort on the front leg**
- **Dumbbell on working side**

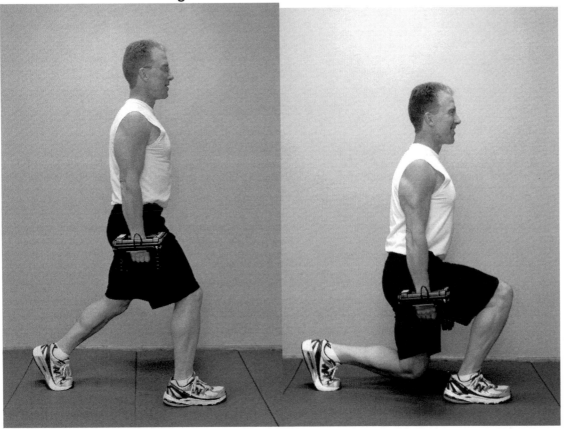

Finish position:
- **Vertical torso**
- **Shoulders and hips parallel**
- **Weight stays on front leg**

Step forward far enough that the rear heel comes off the floor. The bottom position should approximate right angles at the knees. Keep your weight and effort on the front leg; the back leg is for stability. In this version, keep your torso vertical; this creates zero moment arm for the glutes, and emphasizes the quadriceps and hamstrings. The staggered stance also means that the deep muscles on each side of the hip work stabilize each leg independently, more so than with the conventional squat or leg press. If you're going to add weight, hold a dumbbell on either the working side alone or one dumbbell in each hand: definitely do not use a barbell. My preference is to do all reps on one leg, then switch, so that you set your position once. If you switch legs each rep, you'll have to reset your posture between reps, giving you more rest within the set.

REVERSE LUNGE

- **Step back with the non-working leg.**
- **Lean your torso forward with a stable back.**
- **Use your front leg to drive back to standing.**

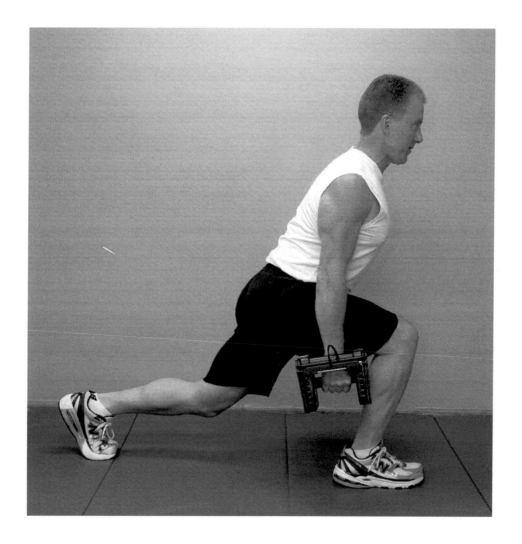

In the Split Squat, you step forward(lunge) to get in position, and then you squat with a vertical torso, to focus on the quadriceps and hamstrings. The Reverse Lunge rearranges the moment arms to emphasize the glutes. You step one foot to the rear, keeping your weight and effort on the front leg. As you lean your torso forward, your hip moves away from your center of gravity, creating a moment arm for the glutes. In this and the Split Squat, whether you alternate sets for each leg, or alternate reps within the set is a matter of preference. It is more important to control and stabilize during the set, than it is to adhere to a particular set/rep scheme.

HEEL RAISE

Start position:
- Bent ankles
- Slightly bent knees
- Bodyweight on the metatarsal break

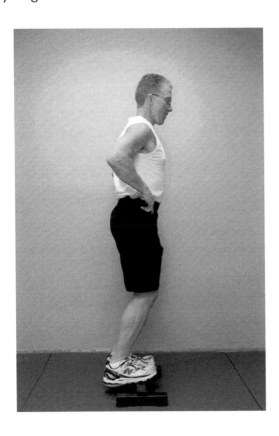
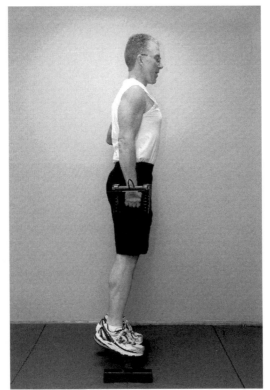

Finish position:
- **Heels lifted**
- **Straight knees**
- **Bodyweight stays on the break**

The conventional "calf" raise is deceptive in terms of the amount of weight and reps handled. By shifting your bodyweight, you're able to turn your calf and ankle into a "wheelbarrow" and use the leverage advantage simply to put up gaudy numbers without effectively challenging your calves. The extra weight and reps still has to be supported (at least) by the small structures of the foot (and maybe the spine if you load that way). In this version, you shift your weight to feel the pressure on the metatarsal break ("ball of the foot"); this minimizes any leverage for the calf. The soleus works with any heel raise, as it attaches the shin to the foot. To work the gastrocnemius efficiently, you want to move from "stretched at the heel and shortened at the knee", to "shortened at the heel and stretched at the knee", which avoids insufficiencies. If you need additional weight, hold the dumbbell on the side of the working calf. Holding the weight on the off side makes balancing more difficult on the lower back without extra challenge to the calf.

CONGRUENT CHIN-UP

Start position:
- **Parallel or EZ grip**
- **Shoulders down and back**
- **Lean your torso back**

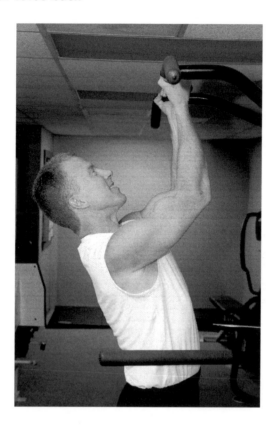 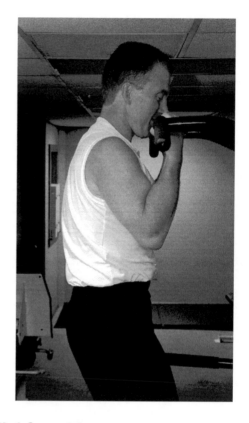

Finish position:
- **Pull into a "crunch"**
- **Shoulders stay down and back**
- **Elbows stay in front of torso**

A more precise form in the chin-up can save your shoulders and more efficiently work the latissimus dorsi. The cleanest path for your arm to move overhead is somewhere between parallel upper arms and arms fully in line to the sides; i.e. between shoulder width and wide grip. Exactly where is based on the individual. Ideally, you would choose between an EZ bar grip, a parallel grip, or movable grips, (to avoid hand and wrist strain), slightly wider than shoulder width (to avoid shoulder strain). In addition, you want to avoid loading the shoulder with the upper arms too much greater than 90 degrees of shoulder flexion. This is the joint angle of peak torque for the lats. Above this, none of the major upper body muscles are positioned near their strong positions, so all your weight would be hanging through your shoulders, being held together by the muscles of the rotator cuff—or not, in which case, the soft tissues in the shoulder are getting the brunt of it. Keeping your shoulders down and back during the chin engages the larger trapezius, and leaning back at the start keeps the latissimus near its strongest position. At the top, allow a slight crunch in the midsection: since the lats connect the upper arm to the pelvis, this is a natural response to their effort.

STRAIGHT-ARM PULLDOWN

- **Shoulders down and back**

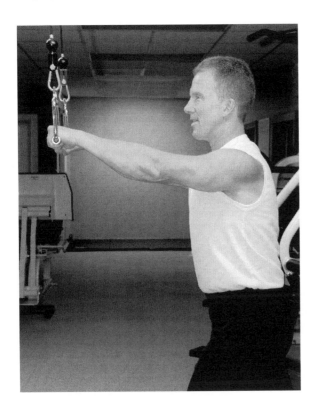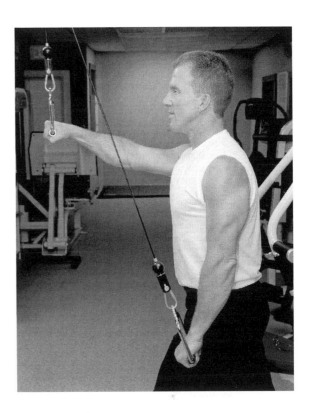

- **One leg forward for stability**   **Both or alternate arms**

This is a far safer version of pullover exercise, whether with free weights or station. A staggered stance keeps you from pulling yourself towards the cable. The weight stack should just be engaged at the start position, i.e. with your arms straight in front and parallel to the floor, you should be supporting the load. There should be right angles between the cable and your arms, and your arms and your torso to match the sticking point with the lats' strongest position. Ideally, you have individual handles, as shown, but either a straight bar or rope is adequate.

ONE-ARM ROW

- Bodyweight spread between your feet and the hand on the bench.
- Shoulders and hips parallel to floor.
- Pull the dumbbell, your elbow, and your shoulder, towards your hip.

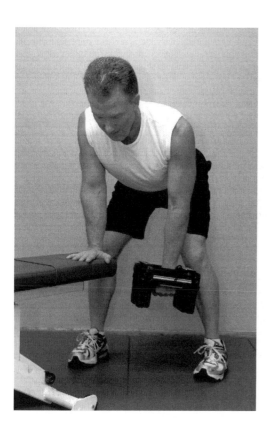 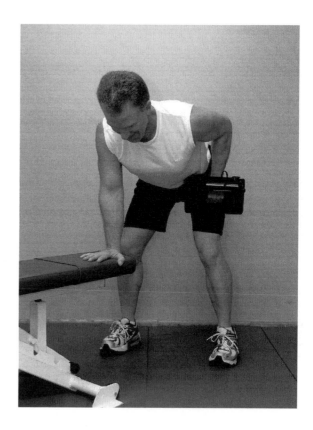

- Avoid "starting the lawn mower" or twisting the spine; also avoid sagging the shoulder at the bottom.
- Bend your knees to return the dumbbell to the floor.

Not an effective exercise for the latissimus, as the sticking point is well past the lats' strongest position; but very effective for the trapezius and other scapula retractors. Keep your knees bent slightly, allowing you to maintain the curve in the lumbar spine. The tripod stance puts equal weight on your feet and hand to minimize twisting around the spine. To load the muscles around the spine appropriately, rather than twisting against resistance, concentrate on resisting the twist. To start and finish, maintain the curves in your spine and level shoulders, and do a partial squat to lift/return the dumbbell to the floor.

SEATED ROW

- **Shoulders down and back**
- **Brace with the legs and trunk**
- **Hold the shoulders in place while you pull with the elbows**

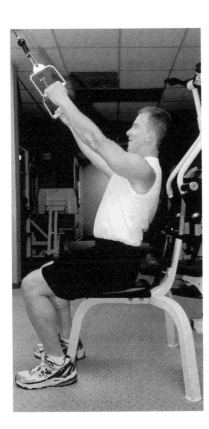 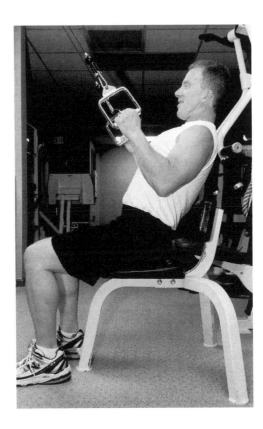

Demonstrated on the Nautilus Freedom Trainer. Make sure your cable column has a broad enough base so you don't pull it over on you; not all equipment designs can accommodate this angle of pull. Be sure to pull both your elbows and shoulders back. Unlike the Chin-Up, do not pull into a crunch at the finish; maintain an upright back posture to encourage pulling back the scapulae. As with any Row, the resistance is less effective in working the lats' than the trapezius and muscles around the spine. This version works spine extension more so than the One-Arm Row, which resists spine rotation.

CONGRUENT PUSH-UP

- Handles in line with the lower border of pectorals.

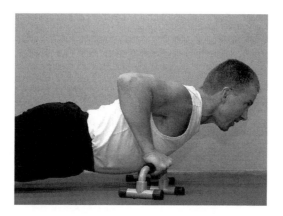

- Handles slightly wider than shoulder width.

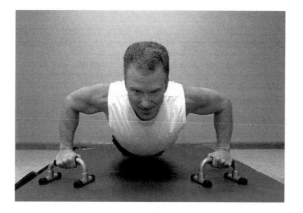

- Elbows unlocked at the finish

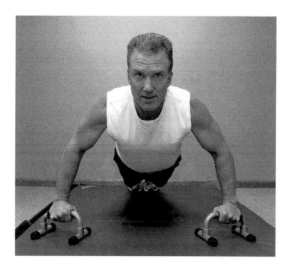

As with the Chin-Up, more precise form is more efficient and can minimize shoulder strain. The exact position of your hands should be based on your individual, pain-free range, but there are some general considerations. With your hands wider than shoulder-width, your center of gravity opposes bringing your arms together (function of the pectorals) more than straightening the elbow. Placing your hands directly in line with the shoulders (pure adduction) is hard on the shoulder joint, however, so a hand position approximately in line with the bottom of the sternum/lower border of the pectorals is a good starting point. Angled handles take some strain off the wrists, by not forcing your hands flat against the floor, bending your wrists back. Direct the pressure to the heels of your hands, not the palms. You can also adjust the way the handles line up with each other, not necessarily in line (barbell style), but whichever way is easiest on your joints.

When bodyweight becomes too easy, there has been a tendency to make push-ups harder by increasing the range around the shoulder (between chairs, blocks, dipping bars, etc.) This is a mistake: it is only harder on the shoulder joint, since there is no knee cap in the shoulders. A better option to increase your effort is with manual (partner) resistance, or a weighted vest, or with elastic cables designed for this purpose, while using the same specific range of loading.

VERTICAL CHEST PRESS

- **Use the vertical handles.**

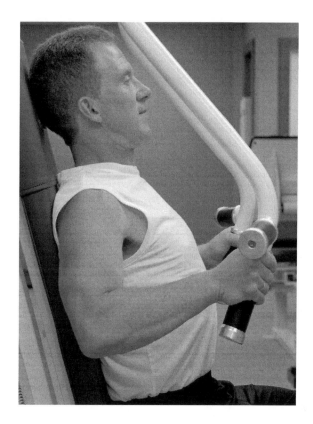

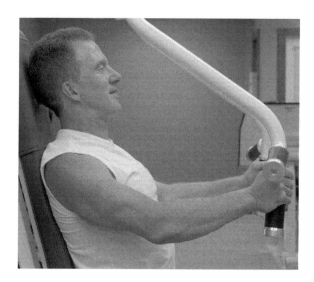

- **Do not load the shoulder behind the torso.**

- **Elbows unlocked at the finish**

Push-ups work well around bodyweight capability; but if you have to use significantly less or more than your bodyweight, push-ups aren't very adaptable. While the machine isn't as challenging to the core as the push-up, the machine can be more specific to challenging the pushing muscles of the upper body. You should still mimic the limb positions of the push-up, and maintain your overall posture during the set. Most machine designs pander to the idea of an extreme stretch, so you may not be able to set the bottom position to prevent it. If you can, set the machine so the weight stack touches as the back of your arms are about to break the plane of your back, or short of that, if that is where your pain-free range is. If the machine can't be set, while looking straight ahead, keep your hands in your peripheral vision during the set. If you can't see your hands, you may be overstretching the shoulder. At you push the handles away from you, stop just short of locking your elbows, and don't hunch your shoulders forward or crunch. The main function of the pectorals is adduction of the arms. Rolling your shoulders forward is done by the much smaller serratus, and since the pectorals attach to the sternum, not the pelvis, crunching only flattens the lumbar curve, adding spine involvement with no added benefits.

INCLINE SIDE RAISE

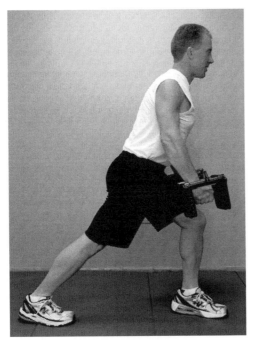
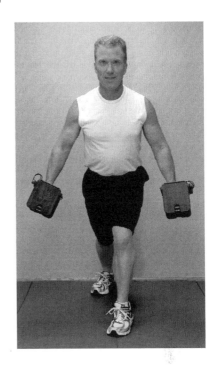

- One leg forward to support the back

  - Don't allow the dumbbells to rest directly below the shoulders

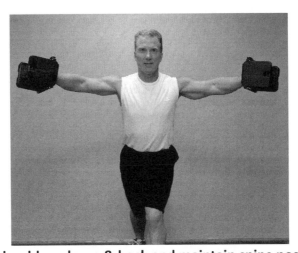

- Keep shoulders down & back and maintain spine posture

Positioning your torso forward at about 60 degrees improves the side raise in two ways. The side deltoid is positioned to work directly against the vertical line of the resistance and the incline encourages external rotation, avoiding any impingement. Unfortunately, without a machine with a specific cam, it's awkward to match muscle and resistance torque with free weights. Free weights in this exercise are mechanically most difficult in the top position, while the deltoids are strongest at about 60 degrees of abduction (arms slightly away from the torso); so much of the side raise is too easy. One way to minimize this effect is to not lower the dumbbells directly beneath the shoulders (avoiding a zero moment arm) during the set. Be sure to maintain your spine posture.

STANDING REAR DELT

- Stabilize the lower body and trunk
- Straight (but not locked out) elbow
- At the start the band should be parallel to your shoulders and taut

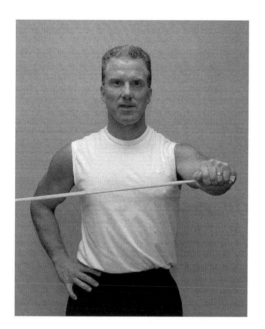 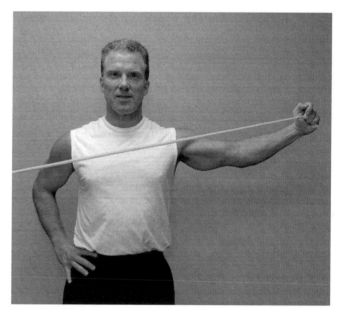

First make sure the elastic is anchored securely. Stand so your hips and shoulders are parallel to the line of the elastic at the start position. Stand far enough away from the anchor that you feel some resistance with your arm raised to shoulder height, pointing straight ahead, palm down. Stabilize your lower body and trunk, and pull your arm from 12:00 (straight ahead) to 3:00 (to the side), into external rotation. As the elastic stretches and comes closer to you, the moment arm is shrinking, offsetting the increased resistance from the stretched elastic. Keep your shoulder down and back, and resist twisting through the trunk during the set.

STANDING EXTERNAL ROTATION

- Stabilize the lower body and trunk
- Elbow locked at a right angle
- At the start the band should be parallel to your shoulders and taut

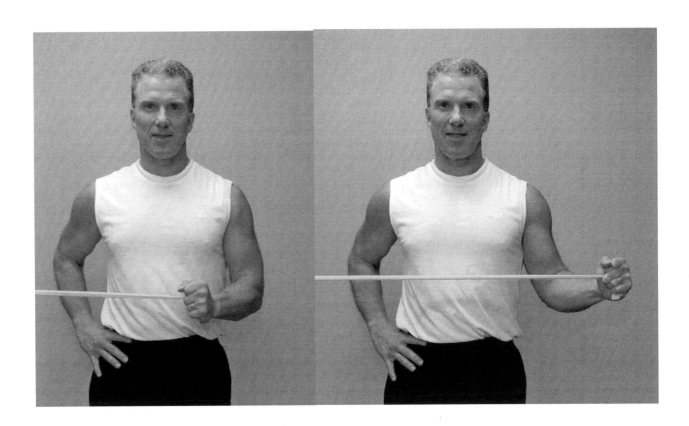

First make sure the elastic is anchored securely. Stand so your hips and shoulders are parallel to the line of the elastic at the start position. Stand far enough away from the anchor that you feel some resistance in the start position, with your forearm angled across your ribcage. Stabilize your lower body and trunk, and pull your arm from 2:00 (across the ribcage) to 10:00 (to the side). As the elastic stretches and comes closer to you, the moment arm is shrinking, offsetting the increased resistance from the stretched elastic. Your forearm should move about 90 degrees, with your upper arm rotating in place like an axle. In the finish, your forearm should be well short of pointing directly to the side.

CONGRUENT CURL

- **Split stance, to support the back**
- **Alternate arms**
- **Palm up for the biceps, thumb up for the brachioradialis of the forearms**

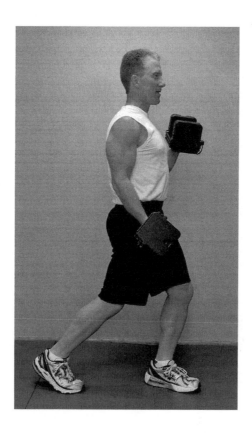

The conventional barbell curl is eventually hard on the elbows and back. The palms-up (supinated) grip that the bar dictates strains the elbow due to the "carrying angle", which guides the hand towards the center when you bend your elbow with palms up. You relieve this strain by coming out of full supination, which dumbbells allow. As the bar moves forward, your center of gravity moves forward also, which should pitch you face first to the ground. It doesn't, because the deep muscles of the back contract, shifting your head and shoulders away from the barbell to help you keep your balance. However, this now puts extra strain on your back. The split stance broadens your base of support, and alternating dumbbells means less weight moving forward. Both aspects combine to be less challenging to your center of gravity and so to minimize back involvement. Free weights are effective at matching muscle and resistance torque, especially if you avoid locking out (moving the dumbbells either directly above or below the elbow).

INCLINE CURL

- **Adjust the bench so you lean back into the seat**
- **Keep the dumbbells away from directly over or under the elbows**
- **Palm up for biceps, thumb up for brachioradialis of the forearms**

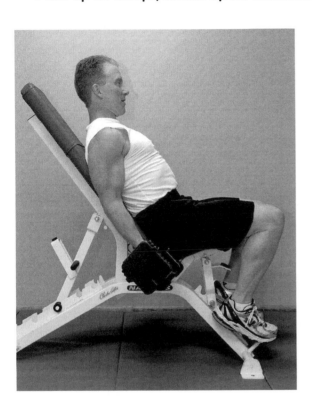 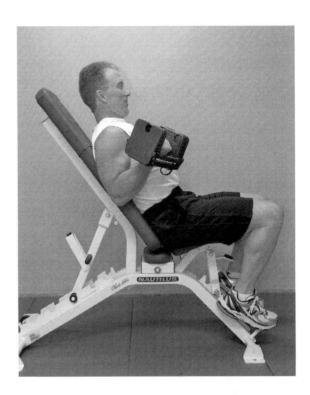

A classic conventional exercise that is perfectly congruent for the biceps, elbow, and back. The dumbbells allow for any degree of supination, from neutral to full. The broad base means that as the dumbbells move forward, your center of gravity isn't disrupted, and the incline position means the muscles around the spine don't necessarily try to move the spine, since your head and shoulders are already away from the weights. As with other exercises, keeping the weights away from zero moment arm (either directly under or directly over the elbow) eliminates the dead zone and becomes a close match for torque. To emphasize the forearm (brachioradialis), keep the dumbbells in the neutral position (hammer curls). To position the biceps to be the prime mover, you should come away from neutral towards a more (not necessarily full) supinated position (shown).

TRICEPS PUSH-UP

- **Handles directly under sternum**

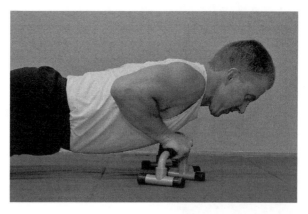

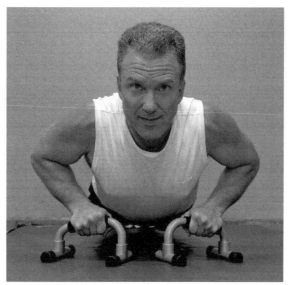

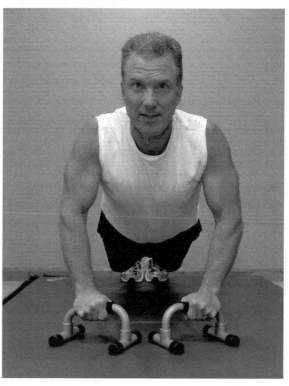

- **Space between hands shoulder width or narrower**

- **Elbows unlocked at the finish.**

As with regular push-ups, the exact hand position should be based on avoiding strain and not just the perceived muscle isolation. Since your center of gravity moves during the exercise (as opposed to dumbbells, for example), it's difficult to position the moment arms to isolate one joint. Generally, though, with your hands closer than shoulder-width, your center of gravity opposes the triceps' action, elbow extension, more so than the pectorals' (shoulder adduction). To protect the shoulder, placing the hands in line with the sternum is a good starting point. The only difference between this push-up and the Congruent Push-Up would be the width of the hand position; all the other suggestions apply.

PRESSDOWN

- **Individual handles**
- **Only move the forearm**
- **Hands end slightly outside hips**

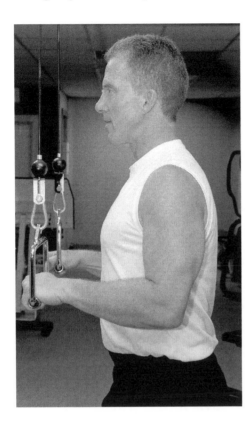 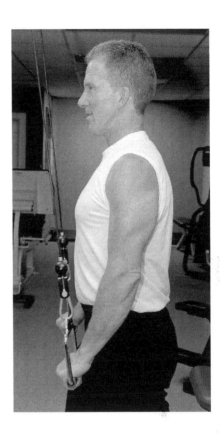

Subtle changes make this exercise much easier on your wrists and elbows than conventional instructions. Doing the exercise one arm at a time, or with independent handles, avoids the binding in the hands and wrists and allows pure elbow extension, without joint complications causing the elbows to flare, turning the exercise into a bad bench press. At the start, you should engage the weight stack with right angles at the cable, forearm, and elbow, with the elbow at your side. This matches the sticking point with the triceps' strongest position. You then straighten the elbow, pulling the handle to the side of your hips/thighs. If your upper arm moves at all, it should move forward as your elbow straightens, taking advantage of the "sawing action". Individual handles, as shown, individual ropes, or an E-Z bar allow the wrist and elbows to avoid the binding that comes with a straight bar or short rope.

TRUNK EXTENSION

- Feet apart for stability
- Start with bent knees, hips, and stable spine
- Finish with straight knees, hips, and spine; but short of the end range

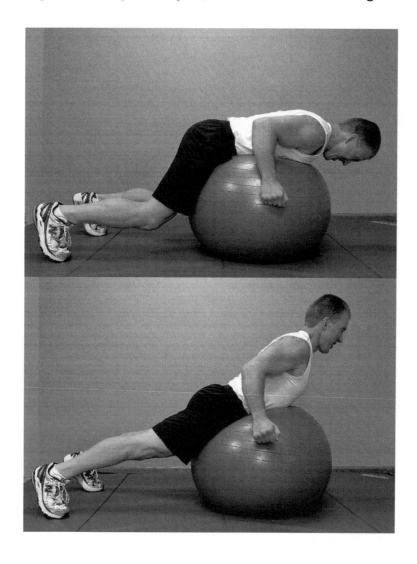

Loading the muscles around the spine is easy. Barbell squats, all versions of the deadlift and row, Olympic lifts, "lower back machines", hyperextensions on the floor and off benches, and kettlebells all unavoidably involve the erector spinae and the "transversospinalis" muscle groups (semispinalis, multifidis, and rotatores).

They also unavoidably involve the discs and connective tissue, which is where the risk lies. A normally curved spine puts even pressure on the discs; the curve of the overall spine comes from the non-symmetrical shape of each individual vertabrae, stacked on each other, separated by the (flat) discs. Maintaining the curves in the spine protects the discs and muscles. Twisting the spine, and exagerating or flattening the curves in the spine, while exerting force, or under load, or with excessive repetitions, deforms the discs and strains the muscles, potentially leading to herniations, spasms, arthritis, etc.

There are several concerns with most "back" exercises. First, you don't really know what is happening at the level of the discs, at least until symptoms occur. The consequence of mis-loading the discs may not be immediate; it may just accelerate long term wear. You may voluntarily try to keep your back tight during a squat, deadlift, (etc.), you may appear as if you are, but the weight is definitely trying to bend your spine forward. Since you can't see into the spine, you don't really know if each of the deep muscles is holding the vertabra in place; they may not be, creating the impingement/herniation, just not yet at a noticeable level. You may squat/deadlift/etc. for years, then tie your shoes and "throw your back out".

You may, however, notice immediately if one of those muscles overstretches and goes into spasm, so the second concern is whether the muscle action for the exercise is appropriate. Only a small part of the erector spinae attaches to the pelvis; the rest attaches vertabrae to ribs (and again a small part to the head). The rest of the muscle groups connect vertabrae to vertabrae in various directions. Combine the short muscle connections, with the fact of the deep muscles having no room to hypertrophy (so any strength displayed comes from static strength), with the fact of the non-twisted curves being the safe position for the discs, with the fact of limited flexion-extension in the lumbar spine, and it strongly suggests that the function of these muscles is to prevent motion more so than to create it. An appropriate exercise would require the muscles to prevent spine flexion more than create extension, and to prevent rotation more than create it.

In order to do that, the pelvis has to be able to follow the spine. If the pelvis is locked in place, say by locking out your knees, and then bending forward, the hamstrings go taut, lock the pelvis in place, and so any upper body motion happens through the spine, not the hip joint. The more your torso moves forward, the more taut the hamstrings, the more the lumbar curve flattens or reverses, the more bad stress to the discs and muscles trying to control the vertabrae. Any exercise to benefit the back has to avoid this.

The demonstrated exercise starts with the knees and hips bent, with a stabilized torso over the ball. The horizontal orientation means the weight of your torso is trying to pull your spine into flexion. The bent knees and hips allows the pelvis to tilt forward and maintains the lumbar curve. If you were to try to lift the torso with the knees bent and the pelvis tilted forward, the erector spinae would pull the lumbar into an exaggerated curve until the bony spines stopped the motion (and pinch the discs). Instead, you move from bent knees/bent hips to straight knees/straight hips, while holding the back posture. The hamstrings and glutes are the prime movers, pulling on the pelvis, while the erector spinae (and quadratus lumborum) hold the pelvis to the spine, and the deep muscles hold the spine posture. The overall effect is to raise the torso approximately in line with the legs, but short of the maximum arch of the spine. The side-to-side instability of the ball requires the muscles to prevent rotation. If a bench is used, ideally, it would allow the same knee/hip coordination. If it doesn't, it's more important to start with the bent knees/forward torso to protect the lumbar curve, than to lock the knees at the finish. Simply make a point of stopping the upward movement before exaggerating the lumbar curve.

TWISTING CRUNCH

- **Feet apart for stability**
- **The ball supports the lumbar curve**
- **Move one shoulder towards the opposite hip, without lifting the lower back off the ball**

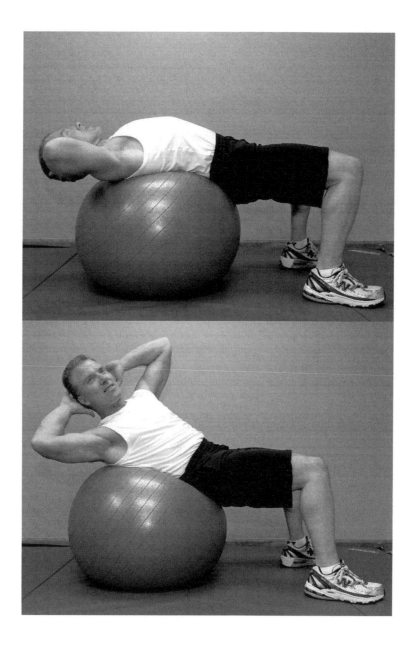

Exercises for the sides and front of the trunk can also risk the lumbar spine. The conventional sit-up and leg raises fell out of favor, to be replaced by versions of the crunch, which turn out to have their own issues. Since the attachments, shapes, and sizes of the front and side muscles are significantly different from the deep back muscles, they need specific positioning and actions, but the exercises also need to protect the discs by maintaining the curves of the spine.

The muscles on the side and front are the external and internal obliques, rectus abdominus, and the transverse abdominis, all of which are more superficial than the transversospinalis groups. Unlike the tvs groups, which connect vertebrae to vertebrae, the obliques and rectus generally connect ribs to pelvis in various directions. A static contraction supports the spine by preventing movement around the trunk, keeping the deep muscles from being overpowered in stabilizing the spine. An active contraction brings the ribs towards the hips (and vice versa), which is where the complications are.

The issue with old school sit-ups and leg raises is that other muscles are involved in bending the body in half. Part of the quadriceps (rectus femoris) connects hip to leg, so while it (and multiple other hip flexors) can pull the front of the thigh towards the pelvis, it also pulls the front of the pelvis towards the thigh. This creates an "anterior pelvic tilt", which can exaggerate the lumbar curve, especially during leg raises. With sit-ups, while the "abs" pull ribs to pelvis, and the hip flexors pull the pelvis towards the quadriceps, neither raises the torso off the floor. This is done by the psoas, a deep muscle that connects the femur to the lumbar spine. The pull of the psoas, plus the anterior tilt, further increases the lumbar curve.

The crunch appeared to be the solution. However, overdoing the crunch, moving to the end point of bending the spine, reverses the lumbar curve, also an issue for disc health. At this point, you feel a cramping sensation, which is commonly accepted as a sign of an effective ab work, but is actually active insufficiency. By itself, the cramping isn't necessarily negative, just not productive. The issue is the stress on the discs from reversing the lumbar curve. This also happens if the pelvis is free to move during the crunch: the same action that pulls the ribs to the pelvis pulls the other way, too, creating a "posterior pelvic tilt" (the back side of the pelvis tilting towards the hamstrings). Contracting the hamstrings and glutes during ab exercise also creates the posterior tilt. By themselves, the anterior and posterior tilts aren't necessarily to be avoided; but load, effort, speed, and high repetitions puts extra strain on the discs.

In the demonstrated exercise, the feet are apart to provide a stable base; as you progress, you can move the feet closer together to make it more challenging. Hips are slightly in front of the center of the ball, to avoid an extreme anterior tilt and excessive lumbar curve. Stay in the midrange of possible movement over the ball; you want the ball to support the lumbar curve, not reverse the thoracic curve. Start well short of fully arched over the ball. The bent knees will keep some tension on the quads, but also consciously tighten the quads in a static contraction to help lock the pelvis in place . Avoid tightening the hamstrings and glutes. Only lift your shoulders off the ball, towards the opposite hip, again stopping well short of the maximum bend in the spine. Hands on the head is optional, if you find your neck straining before your abs. Don't pull on the head; feel the weight of your head in your hands. Crossing your arms across your chest removes the weight of your arms from the load; if you do this, keep a tight neck without thrusting with the chin or letting your head fall back.

7. The Congruent Context

Just so there is no misunderstanding: the point of the Congruent Exercises isn't the names of the exercises, or the brand name on the equipment, or whether you use dumbbells or machines or elastic or swiss balls or bodyweight or any particular form of resistance. The main point is the Effective Range of Loading, the joint movements and postures that the most fundamental aspects of anatomy and biomechanics indicate are safe to load, and that for the most part, coordinate both resistance torque and muscle torque, to make for a more efficient exercise.

None of which guarantees an injury-free, or ailment-free, experience. Accidents happen: you can always drop a dumbbell on your foot. Mistakes happen: you get motivated for an extra rep, you put some extra "body English", a muscle goes into spasm. Pre-existing conditions pre-exist: you may have an old injury from sports, or overuse condition from work, and it flares up as you exercise. Undiagnosed inflammations catch up with you: the symptoms of arthritis, bursitis, tendinitis, etc., which have accumulated over years, suddenly become noticeable. And if you regularly load your joints outside the range of proper joint function, as described in the most basic anatomy and biomechanics texts, you run the risk of accelerating all those issues, and of the exercise program itself creating new ones.

I suspect there are a few people who will disagree with that last, who have a rationale for loading the extremes. (OK, maybe more than a few.) They'll insist that they've "trained this way for years and never had a problem", when what they mean is that they haven't had an acute injury. Or that your body will "get used to" loading the extreme motions, that it will somehow adapt outside of conventional biomechanics, which ignores the cumulative effect of wear and tear over time. Or that you have to take great risks to get great rewards-whatever that may be in the exercise context. Or what doesn't kill you makes you stronger. If they are happy with their training, I'm not going to try to convince them otherwise, although I've found they become much more receptive after the aches and pains start.

For me, however, there is no alternative. Call me crazy, but exercise is intended to benefit the body, not risk it. Simply work as hard as your motivation allows within the safe ranges, on the resistance source of your choice, and whatever benefits you would have gotten while exceeding those ranges you'll get with much less risk.

Here are some suggestions on how to apply the material.

Reset your weights. When you adjust your ranges, you'll probably have to change your working weight, depending on the exercise. If you're used to locking out, it may decrease. But, if you've been trying to load the extreme ranges, it may increase, because you're no longer trying to load the weak positions. There's no simple rule of thumb, so reduce the weight and practice the movement until you find a working weight.

Breathing. Remember to. Start with the conventional advice to exhale as you lift and inhale as you lower the weight. As the set gets harder and you want to breathe faster, don't worry about coordinating the breath with the lift, just breathe as you need. Don't hold your breath, which seems to be a common response to the harder work. Holding breath will feel more stable, because of the air column that forms in front of the torso, but it's better to stabilize with your muscles.

"Bracing yourself" vs. substitution vs. cheating. While "bracing" is not the clinically accurate term, you should actively tighten all your muscles during a set, not just the targets of the exercise for two reasons. First, a moderate static contraction will use the fixation function of muscle to prevent unwanted shifts in posture, which will both protect the spine and provide the stable platform for the prime movers. Second, from the perspective of effort, outside of the exercise field, it's pretty established that engaging muscles beyond the prime movers in a task is associated with more effort from the prime movers. You don't want to engage them so much that they try to substitute for the targets of the exercise, nor do you want to actively move the weight (cheat) with the other muscles. Either may add numbers to your routine, but you lose control of the effects of the exercise.

Pacing the repetition and the set. Think "lift-pause-resist" rather than "heave-swing-drop" during each rep. On weight stacks, as you return the weight, think of putting a cup in a saucer rather than slamming down a shot glass. An exact time count for each rep doesn't work because of the different distances covered in each exercise, so aim for effort on both aspects of the rep, without momentum either up or down. A time count for the set, however, may be helpful, so you can concentrate on the movement and not counting reps.

Ending the set. You're lifting-pausing-resisting, the targeted muscles may be burning or just feeling less energetic than at the start, you're maintaining a tight posture without substitution or cheating. Deciding to end the set is more an issue of motivation than an exact, objective marker. If the form breaks (substitution or cheating), consider correcting it one time and try again. If it breaks a second time, end the set. If the form doesn't break, you'll have to decide how hard to push. A window of 30 to 90 seconds seems to be an accepted duration for strength training, so try to maintain the form for at least 30 seconds, with a weight that encourages you to run out of energy/motivation before 90 seconds. This is roughly 6 to 20 reps, depending on the exercise. Use seconds or reps, whichever you prefer. You may notice a "sweet spot" for different exercises. At the last repetition, don't collapse under the weight; still maintain the postures and control as you return the weight.

Advanced techniques. The highly motivated individual may reach this point and feel "it isn't enough". The traditional approach is to then thrash, heave, gnash teeth, bulge eyes, and pop blood vessels, which tends to distract from maintaining posture and avoiding substitution. If you are motivated to go past the end of the set, but not the traditional way, several advanced techniques work well with this approach.

As far as muscles are concerned, all advanced techniques deplete more energy and add more byproducts of contraction ("burn"), usually by extending the set. The issue is which techniques are most manageable with regard to protecting the joints. Rest-pause and supersets are the most efficient, and effective at maintaining joint stabilization. With rest-pause, after your last rep, put the weight down, take 3 deep breaths (just as a way of gathering yourself), reset your posture, and do at least one more positive rep, followed by the slowest negative possible. With supersets, the change in exercises gives you the chance to reset, especially with opposing muscle groups. Two different exercises for the same muscle group also works; while the prime movers are the same, the stabilizing pattern changes, so you continue to work the prime movers past the end of the first set.

Of course, if the basic format isn't "enough", you can always add a second or third work set of the original exercise. However, any set-extending technique requires extra recovery, and it's questionable whether using them delivers more benefit. Your priority should be the basic set format, with advanced techniques used for novelty.

Routines. The best routine is the one you do regularly. If you're already comfortable with how you've organized your exercises, trips to the gym, equipment, etc., simply changing the ranges to those demonstrated should be easier on your joints going forward (subject to whatever you've done in the past). If your routine isn't working for you, here is a structure I use with home and studio clients.

Exercise order. Chest and Back, Lower Body, Arms, Trunk. Include Shoulders with either with Chest and Back or Arms. If you prefer to do them all in one workout, keep the order but rotate the lead group of exercises. For example, Monday starts with Chest and Back, Thursday starts with Lower Body, the next Monday Arms. If doing them all in one day is too much, split the routine in approximately the same order, so that if circumstances dictate two days in a row, there is minimal overlap.

Basic Stage. In Basic, you are relearning how to do the exercises and finding your working weight. Start with at least two sets of six reps, with the first deliberately light to practice the form. Add weight each set, keeping the specific form, until you find the weight that encourages you to stop in the 30-90 second window. This doesn't have to happen all in one workout; take as many as you need to lock in the form. For the exercises that don't use weights, end the first set well before you want to and push the effort on the second set. Move to the next stage when your form is set and you are pushing the second set hard in that 30-90 second range.

Intermediate Stage. Now you will work on more intense effort for each set. Do at least a ten-minute overall warm-up, and go right into the work sets. Your work sets are under control, you're not putting the joints in vulnerable positions, and you're not thrashing at the end of the set, so the practice set is optional. Occasionally, pick one or two exercises per workout to do an additional work set, rest-pause, or superset, based on what you think you need. Aim to keep any rest periods to 30 seconds as you want to be recovered enough to exert another serious effort on the next set. If you prefer overall routines, do two separate routines alternating exercises, rather than one longer routine, to avoid feeling too depleted. Split routines, if you keep the total number of sets low, allow you to concentrate on the effort for each exercise without interfering with later exercises. This may be the most productive and sustainable stage of training, that you stay in for most of your training year.

Advanced Circuits. If you've gone through the previous two stages, you know the joint-friendly form and how to exert safely on each exercise. Now you combine these with minimal rest between sets for a greater overall metabolic challenge. You will rush between exercises and push each exercise, just with more control than if you just jumped into a class or dvd and tried to keep up. Set your timer for 1:00 repeats, assemble your exercises for a whole body routine, and aim to do 30 sets in 30 minutes, all in proper form and effort. This will take more out of you than you're used to, but you're saving it for a two week stretch when you're particularly motivated. Aim for 2 or 3 sessions each week for that two weeks, then drop back to the Intermediate stage.

<u>Sample Workouts</u>
Basic Home Workout (whole body)(once or twice/week)
- 10:00 Overall Warm-Up (walk, bike, treadmill, skip rope, etc.)
- :30 rest between sets
- 6 reps per set; the first set light, the second heavier, except where noted
1. Congruent Push-up: first set, 6 reps; second set, work towards 12 reps
2. One-Arm Row: alternate arms for each set
3. Incline Side Raise
4. Reverse Lunge: alternate legs each rep; first set 6 reps each, second set, up to 10 each
5. Congruent Curl: alternate arms each rep
6. Triceps Push-up: (same scheme as above)
7. Trunk Extension: first set, 10 reps; second, work towards 20
8. Twisting Crunch: alternate each rep; first set 6 each side, second set, work towards 10 each

Basic Home Workout (two day split)(two sessions/week): first four on day one, last four on day two.
Basic Home Workout (three day split)(3x/week): new exercises*
    Monday: Congruent Push-up, Row, Side Raise,*Standing Rear Delt
    Wednesday: *Hip Belt Squat, Reverse Lunge, *Split Squat
    Friday: Curl, Triceps Push-up,*External Rotation, Trunk, Crunch

Intermediate Home Workout (sample "extra" schemes for each group)(see text for program)
- 10:00 warm-up
- Congruent Push-up, up to 1:30, followed by 2 rest-pause reps
- One-Arm Row, each hand alternating, no rest, 12 reps, 10 reps, 8 reps
- Split Squat, alternate sets, 10x3, no rest between legs/sets
- Reverse Lunge, alternate legs, with dumbbells, Trunk Extension x 20, Twisting Crunch x 20
- Side Raise, 12 reps, followed by one rest-pause; Standing Rear Delt, alternating, no rest, 15, 12, 10. External Rotation, same scheme.
- Congruent Curls, 12 reps (each arm, 24 total), no rest, Triceps Push-ups 90 seconds, repeat cycle

Typical, Individual Training Schedule (mine)
- Monday: 10:00 Arm Bike (Windjammer), 20: Recumbent Bike; Pulldown, Vertical Chest, Row, each for 8-12 reps, no rest. Occasional rest-pause reps on each.
- Tuesday: yoga
- Wednesday: 10:00 Elliptical Trainer, 10:00 Arm Bike; Trunk extension & Twisting crunch, 20x 3 each; Adductor, Abductor, Leg Press, each for 8-12 reps, no rest. Occasional: 3 cycles of 6 reps with the same working weight.
- Thursday: Recreational sports
- Friday: 10:00 Arm Bike, 10:00 Bike ITP, Side Raise, Rear Delt, External Rotation, Curl, Triceps, each for 8-12 reps. Occasional: SR rest-pause. Curl/triceps 3 cycles of 6 reps.
- Saturday and Sunday: Yoga. Recreational sports

Advanced Circuit
Set your stopwatch for 1:00 repeats.
1. Trunk extension
2. Twisting crunch
3. Reverse lunge with dumbbells (alternating legs)
4. Heel Raise with dumbbells
5. Push-up
6. One Arm Row (:30 per arm)
7. Side Raise
8. Split Squat with dumbbells (:30 per leg)
9. Curl
10. Triceps Push-up

The immediate goal is to complete one cycle in ten minutes, with (except for the trunk extension and crunch) a weight that you encourages you to stop near the 1:00 mark. Have the weights prearranged so you can move with no rest from exercise to exercise. Complete 3 cycles per workout.

The first time, underestimate the working weights for the first cycle. Take one minute between cycles. Adjust the weights between cycles so that the second or third cycle gets the right working weight for each exercise for the 1:00 set with no rest.

Over two weeks aim for 3 cycles, with no rest between cycles, with the working weights on the first cycle. The emphasis is on the pace, not the individual effort on each set, so if you need to reduce the weight on the following cycles.

A man came into my studio to have his body fat percentage calculated. In that respect, he was clearly in great shape, but he was bent over with his hand on his lower back and grimacing. What happened to you? "I was doing a (certain brand name) class, working really hard, flipping tires, and my back went out." As I measured what little body fat there was, I told him, look, when your back gets better, train with me a couple of times, I'll show you how to work out just as hard, just as effective, but without injuring your back. And he said, "thanks, but I really like the class, I can't wait to get back. **Look how well it worked**." So this gentleman knew when he got hurt, how he got hurt, and he blamed his back for going out, not the exercise or the pace or previous wear and tear. Clearly, he decided that the cost of getting in admittedly great shape was the risk of injury, and he was OK with that.

For me as a trainer, that's not a choice I'm comfortable making for clients, even if there was some otherwise unattainable benefit to the risky exercises ...and there isn't. One of the benefits they pay for is a safe program. Not just during the session; after the session counts, too.

And for me personally? When I was younger, I did all the exercises, even the ones I now warn about. Back then, I absolutely was not receptive to any well-meaning advice from my physical therapy friends about the long term effects of what I was doing to myself in the gym. Whoops. Mistakes I made in my 20s caught up to me at 40; mistakes I make now, catch up to me later tonight.

Now, the only exercises I do in my own workout and teach to clients are congruent exercises. Best of luck with your training.

8. Recommended Reading

There are three books I recommend for a better understanding of the biomechanics involved with weight training. No affiliate arrangement exists here; feel free to pick them up anywhere.

The Concise Book of Muscles by Chris Jarmey is one of my favorites. It clearly shows individual muscles in context with surrounding muscles and joints, by fading the color of the background structures. I personally use the 2003 version, but there is a second edition available.

Brunstromm's Clinical Kinesiology is a textbook published since 1967 with various contributors. I mainly use this for joint motions, but it also covers the science of muscle, including torque graphs. This is not an easy read; this is a reference text for study. But anyone loading weight to joints, whether their own or someone else's, should study it to see exactly just how joints are supposed to move, especially compared to how they move during exercises. A new version is due in late 2011.

Prime Mover: A Natural History of Muscle by Steven Vogel describes the history of muscle science, both the true and the false. This is an easy read of a complex topic. Vogel is a biologist with several textbooks, including Cat's Paws and Catapults, which is where I saw his explanation of force- or distance-amplifying levers. It's fascinating how so many theories of muscle, many of which were pretty current in the fitness and muscle media, had been clarified many years ago by actual research scientists.

These are three of my favorites, but I cross referenced my readings with other texts; Moment Arm Exercise includes a full list. Any anatomy and biomechanics texts you have access to will confirm how the muscles and joints work, because this is basic science, not interpretation. Just make sure they come from the "medical" or "science" section of the book seller.

For personal trainers, I also like the biomechanics chapters in the old NSCA and ACE Personal Trainer manuals. I used the Essentials of Strength Training and Conditioning 1994 version; the biomechanics chapter by Everett Harman is excellent, which is repeated in at least one subsequent version. The chapter in Personal Trainer Manual: A Resource for Fitness Professionals (1997) from ACE is not as technical but still very good.

While I generally rely on textbooks and not individual studies, two are worth mentioning. "Predictive torque equations for joints of the extremities" from Acta of Bioengineering and Biomechanics, Vol. 4, No. 2, 2002 documents "torque output throughout the range of motion for the human elbow, shoulder, knee, and hip". In other words, it confirms the idea of predictable muscle torque curves. "A Brief Review of Concurrent Activation Potentiation: Theoretical and Practical Constructs", by William P. Ebben, (from the Journal of Strength and Conditioning Research, 2006, 20(4), 985-991, 2006) is a comprehensive explanation of "the acute ergogenic advantage associated with the simultaneous activation of muscles other than the prime mover..." Or, as I like to call it, "bracing yourself" during a set.

These are my sources for the basic science behind Congruent Exercise. The application to actual exercises comes from my own experiences and practice.

9. About the author

Bill DeSimone is an experienced personal trainer, having started in 1983 at the Sports Training Institute in New York City, and now with his own studio, Optimal Exercise, in Cranbury, New Jersey. Along the way, he was certified by both the NSCA and ACE, and worked in corporate, commercial, academic, and private settings.

His own training-induced injuries led to his unique approach, applying textbook biomechanics to conventional free-weight and machine instruction. He first presented this material in a manual, Moment Arm Exercise, in 2004; and since then, in a series of videos on You Tube; at conferences for the NSCA, Club Industry, and High Intensity Training; and as in-services for studio and gym staff.

In addition to one-to-one training in the studio, Bill consults with individual trainees worldwide. Via video, Bill reviews the trainee's form on the equipment available to the trainee and provides an email or telephone consultation.

Bill's presentation, "Basic Biomechanics for Weight Training", is available for conferences and staff training.

Contact Bill at optimalexercise@comcast.net. For new video and updates, subscribe to the Congruent Exercise You Tube channel and Facebook page.

Made in the USA
San Bernardino, CA
31 December 2013